NEAL'S YARD RE

Essential Oils

Methods of extraction • Descriptions • Uses

Psychological profiles • Therapeutic properties

Photographs of plants and oils • Safety data

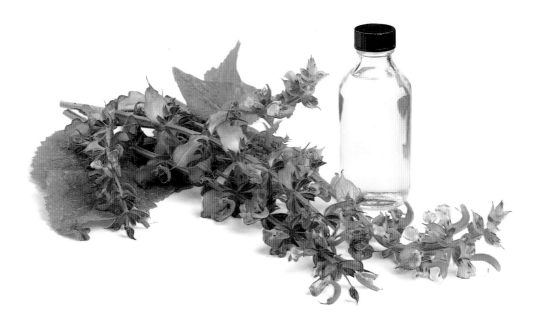

Susan Curtis

AURUM

Author's Acknowledgements

Grateful thanks for their valuable contributions to this book are extended to Arthur Glyn (Bill) Curtis, Sydney Francis, Pauline Hili, Carlo De Paoli, Tamsin Loxley, Lotte Rose and Colin Winter.

First published in the UK in 1996 by

Aurum Press Ltd

25 Bedford Avenue

London WC1B 3AT

Reprinted 1996

Text copyright © Susan Curtis, 1996
Artwork copyright © Haldane Mason, 1996
Copyright © Haldane Mason, 1996

ISBN: 1-85410-413-6

A HALDANE MASON BOOK

Conceived, designed and produced by Haldane Mason, London

Copy Editor: Diana Vowles
Designer: Janet James
Editorial/Production Assistant: Charles Dixon-Spain
Picture Research: Charles Dixon-Spain

Colour reproduction by Regent Publishing Services Ltd
Printed in Hong Kong by Regent Publishing Services Ltd

Picture Acknowledgements

All photographs by Amanda Heywood, with the exception of the following:
A–Z Botanical 47, 91; *Chanel* 53, 109, 123; *J. L. Charmet* 16; *Guerlain* 107; *Images* 12; *Neal's Yard Remedies* 27; *Panos Pictures* 43, 57; *Science Photo Library/G. Hadjo, CNRI* 15, */Geoff Tompkinson* 25.

All illustrations by Debbie Lian Mason, with the exception of the following:
Magda Lazou 8–9, 40–1, 126–7; *Christine Wilson* 73.

Contents

Foreword

Essential oils are an integral part of the Neal's Yard Remedies pharmacopoeia. They are wonderful substances with many different properties, and can be used to benefit both the physical and mental or spiritual sides. Because they are so complex, it is important to have a reliable source of information available when using the oils, so that they can be applied to best effect.

Education and information about our products is an integral part of Neal's Yard Remedies' company ethos. It is particularly important to me, as my background is in education. For six years I helped to run a free school in south London, and although I enjoyed the challenge of teaching in a way that aimed to educate in the true sense of the word, it was an exhausting experience. During this time, I pursued a course in homeopathy. Learning about a system of natural medicine gave me an opportunity to have more involvement in my own health and well-being, and to make informed decisions on issues such as vaccination for my children. It also served to underline how important and empowering it is to be informed about and aware of your own health.

In 1981, I was offered the use of a retail space in Neal's Yard in London's Covent Garden. My frustration in teaching with poor resources and the inability to plan long-term led me to take up this offer with a friend and set up an alternative pharmacy.

For several years I had been impressed by the range and scope of natural medicines available in standard pharmacies in mainland Europe. It seemed that we were missing out in the UK. Aromatherapy in 1981 had hardly been heard of, and having come across the oils, it was important to include them as part of the initial range of products that we provided when the shop opened.

It was clear to me that the use of essential oils was going to be hugely popular for several reasons. The oils themselves convey the very essence of the plant. People with only the most limited sensual experience of the natural world would be delighted by an oil extract. It was as if the oils were the heart and meaning of the plant itself, and here we were, pouring the oils into bottles and selling them.

Not only were essential oils such an opportunity, but the use of them was, too. Massage is a wonderful tool for getting in touch with our own bodies, providing us with the opportunity to give and receive something genuinely real to and from another person. I am convinced that teaching children to massage is something that should be taught from primary school onwards.

It took me some time to realize that essential oils were not only extraordinary, subtle, exciting substances, but they were also very effective. Aromatherapy is a form of natural healing that can be used by every single person; it is entirely accessible. What was needed was really good education into the properties and uses of the oils. Unfortunately, in our society understanding of natural medicines and how they work has been overshadowed by professional administration of drugs and products from the pharmaceutical industry. With these medicines, we can no longer apply our background of knowledge to our own healing processes. The medical profession is trained to take control of people's health. As this attitude has become more prevalent, we find ourselves in a vulnerable and fearful position in respect to our own health and well-being. Increasingly, environmental issues such as stress and pollution are creating a more frightening, disempowering background to health. Aromatherapy provides a way for people to feel more empowered.

In 1984 Susan and I were approached to write a book on medicines. We took up this opportunity, and together with Irene, who also worked in the shop with us, wrote a book on the remedies available from the shop and how people could use them. Although we have always had trained staff behind the counter, it was not always sufficient. People bought things to give to others, or they couldn't always remember what they had been told. With that we completed and published *Neal's Yard Natural Remedies*.

A couple of years later, Susan and I decided to write a book solely on essential oils. What we wanted was not just a book on aromatherapy, but a book that conveyed our love of the oils themselves, their history, where they came from and how the plant was turned into an oil.

Susan and I enjoyed several holidays with the excuse of needing inspiring retreats in which to write the book, but it never really happened. Now Susan has taken our original information and, with the confidence of more than 10 years' expertise and wealth of information, she has written this book.

Essential Oils is well organized, has pictures of all the plants from which the oils come, and Susan's presentation of the constitutional aspects to the oils is thought-provoking and exciting. I am sure it will challenge us to consider oils in a deeper and more intuitive way. As with any form of education, it is what you yourself can contribute to what you learn that is valuable, and not what you have recieved from someone else. I am sure Susan's book will stimulate this process.

Romy Fraser
Managing Director,
Neal's Yard Remedies
London
December 1995

Introduction

Essential oils have been around for millenia, used by many different cultures in a variety of ways – as medicines, in ritual worship, and as cosmetics and perfumes. These are complex substances: each oil is made up of many components which combine to provide its unique physiological and psychological characteristic profile.

This section looks at the properties of essential oils, the methods by which they are extracted, stored and applied, and finishes with information on their safest and most effective uses.

How do Essential Oils Work?

The use of essential oils is one of the fastest-growing forms of natural medicine and is indeed an excellent example of a holistic approach to health – first because essential oils can be used to treat the whole person, body, mind and spirit, and secondly because, unlike conventional medicine, which targets drugs to eradicate a particular disease process, the oils may have a specific action on a disease process but will also support and strengthen the person to throw off the disease. Tea tree oil, for example, will have a direct anti-viral effect on the common cold virus and will also act as an immuno-stimulant, encouraging the body itself to fight the infection.

When looking at the physiological, psychological and spiritual properties of essential oils, bear in mind that these areas are all active simultaneously in an individual. In deciding which essential oil will suit a particular person, choose one that seems indicated on every level for the greatest benefit. Pine oil, for example, is an excellent respiratory antiseptic and decongestant useful for treating bronchitis: it is also stimulating and refreshing for someone feeling tired and worn out, and its psychological profile is for a person who is closed and suffers from feelings of guilt. Using pine will help to relieve a tight chest, revive and refresh the body and help to break down rigidity and guilt so that sensitivity and openness can be better expressed. What this means is that, when choosing an essential oil for yourself or someone else, you need to consider both the specific physical properties of the oil and its more profound characteristics.

MIND AND BODY

An essential oil is composed of individual chemical constituents that in combination provide it with its physiological properties. Rosemary oil, for example, is known to have among its properties those of being antiseptic, antispasmodic, carminative and stimulant. This indicates that it will be useful for treating infections, period pains, flatulence and tiredness.

During the early part of this century, scientists believed that if the chemical constituents thought to be primarily responsible for certain properties were isolated they could be concentrated and rendered even more effective. The constituent could then be synthesized, thus becoming much cheaper to produce than an essential oil. Thymol, for example, a constituent of thyme oil, was used

10

for many years as a disinfectant in hospitals and surgical wards.

It is now becoming more generally appreciated that an essential oil is a very complex combination of hundreds of different constituents and that many of these individual constituents work synergistically together. This means that the combination of constituents as found in an essential oil is more effective and more appropriate in use than an isolated constituent. For example, it has now been found that thyme oil is effective against a much wider variety of pathogens than thymol (its main constituent) and, when used at normal aromatherapy dilutions, is much less likely to be an irritant when applied to the skin. Indeed, most essential oils are better tolerated than their isolated components, which tend to be very much more aggressive in action than a complete essential oil.

Pine, a powerful respiratory antiseptic and decongestant, also revives and refreshes.

This is not to say that essential oils are not toxic – several that are safe to use externally are toxic when taken internally, for example, eucalyptus. Others are safe to use at normal dilutions but are likely to irritate the skin if not diluted before use. There are even some oils that are so toxic they are not available, such as wintergreen. This means that a user of essential oils needs to learn about them in order to employ them with confidence.

An interest in the chemistry of essential oils can be a very useful basis for understanding both the likely properties of an essential oil and any potential toxicity it may have. In France, a system of using essential oils known as clinical aromatherapy has been developed. This is practised by doctors who have acquired a thorough understanding of the physiological properties of essential oils, and who are thus able to prescribe them internally for specific physical ailments.

While the physiological properties are very varied, there are several main areas of action for which essential oils have established their deserved reputation. The first of these is their antiseptic action: all essential oils are antibacterial, although each oil is effective against different pathogens. There have been hundreds of laboratory tests which have shown how just how effective essential oils can be against bacterial, viral, fungal and parasitic infection. Tea tree oil, for example, is effective against streptococcus, gonococcus, pneumococcus, candida albicans, trichomonas vaginalis, herpes simplex, wart virus and scabies, to name but a few. Some clinics,

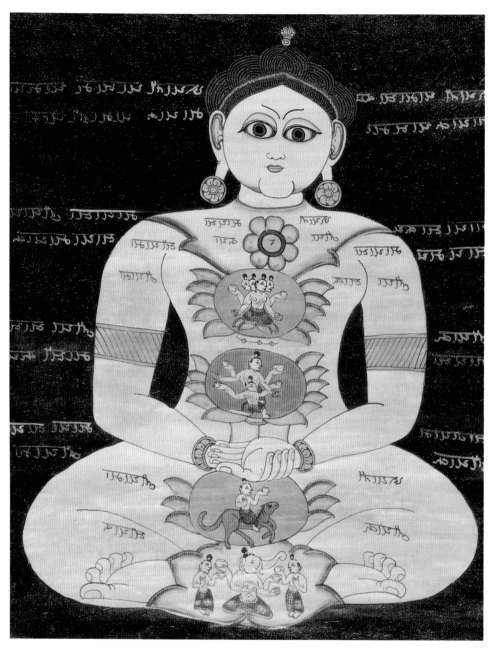

The healing properties of essential oils may be used to improve the body's energy system, or 'prana' as it is known in India.

particularly in France, will culture bacteria taken from a site of infection and expose them to different essential oils to see which oil is most effective against the particular pathogens involved. This process is known as creating an aromatogram. A study in 1971 showed that lemongrass oil was more effective against *Staphyloccocus aureus* (associated with many skin infections) than are penicillin and streptomycin.

Essential oils are known to stimulate the immune response and thereby aid the body in fighting off any infection. It has been shown that all essential oils stimulate phagocytosis, or the ability of white blood cells to dispose of invading bacteria. For example, thyme oil and tea tree oil have been used to benefit people suffering with HIV-related diseases, as they are both strongly antiseptic and excellent immuno-stimulants, as well as being powerful germicides.

Many essential oils have a blood purifying action that works by stimulating the various processes of elimination. This cleansing action means that toxins and metabolic residues which may otherwise lead to a variety of diseases are removed from the system, an effect that is very beneficial in many chronic diseases such as arthritis, as well as helping to reduce cellulite and clear skin problems.

Juniper, a refreshing and detoxifying oil, helps to purify the blood by stimulating the body's elimination processes.

Good examples of detoxifying oils include juniper and rosemary.

A further physiological action of essential oils is upon the endocrine system. This is a group of glands that produce hormones and regulate reproduction, growth, metabolism, our response to stress and the levels of various vital nutrients in the bloodstream. Some essential oils contain phytohormones or 'plant hormones', which act within the body in a similar manner to our own hormones. Phytohormones can reinforce or replace the effects of the corresponding human hormones. Fennel oil, for example, contains a plant oestrogen which stimulates the production of breast milk and can be beneficial in treating symptoms of pre-menstrual tension.

Other essential oils influence the hormone secretion of certain endocrine glands. For example, rosemary oil has a stimulating action on the adrenal cortex, and will help to increase vitality; rose oil has an effect on many of the hormones involved in reproduction and is an excellent treatment for many menstrual and menopausal disorders; while geranium oil tends to have a balancing effect on the endocrine system in general and can

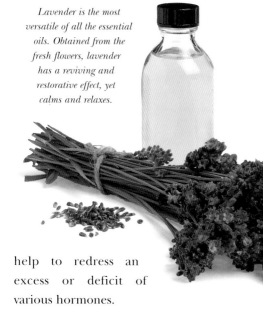

Lavender is the most versatile of all the essential oils. Obtained from the fresh flowers, lavender has a reviving and restorative effect, yet calms and relaxes.

been shown to have a measurable effect on brain activity. Here lies part of the reason why aromatherapy has such wonderful results in the treatment of people who are suffering from stress. Another important factor here is the benefit that will be obtained through receiving a therapeutic massage from an aromatherapist; it is true of many conditions, and stress-related ones especially, that much may be gained from the healing touch of the experienced masseuse.

help to redress an excess or deficit of various hormones.

The endocrine system is a two-way link between our body and our emotions: our hormone secretions affect our moods (as in premenstrual tension), and our moods affect our hormone secretions (as when a sudden shock or fright triggers the secretion of adrenalin). This is why essential oils, by having a therapeutic action on our endocrine system, can have a beneficial action on both our body and our emotions.

Essential oils also have a beneficial effect on our well-being by virtue of their action on the nervous system. Much research has been done to illustrate the sedating or calming properties of certain essential oils such as lavender and neroli, and the stimulating properties of oils such as rosemary. These essential oils have

BODY ENERGY

Another interesting way in which essential oils bring their healing properties to the individual is through their action on what is often called the 'chi' or energy system of the body. The 'chi' as it is known to the Chinese, or 'prana' to the Indians, or 'vital force' in the language of homeopaths, is becoming understood more generally as the electromagnetic field that radiates from the body and gives dynamism and integrity to a living being; when someone dies, their electromagnetic field disintegrates.

In a healthy person, the picture of their electromagnetic field, as shown by Kirlian photography, extends well beyond their physical form and looks vibrant and colourful, whereas in a tired or sick person the electromagnetic field is weak and dull. Essential oils have been shown by the Italian researcher Professor Rovesti and others to have an influence on cellular magnetic fields, and thus their use actually has a direct effect on the dynamic energy system that integrates life itself.

Having considered some of the measurable effects of essential oils, it should be realized that one of the great things about aroma-therapy is that it is about pleasure as well as therapeutics. When choosing an essential oil for a treatment, it is important to make sure its odour is pleasing to the recipient. Part of the benefit of using an essential oil will come from enjoying it, and that is also one of the ways that essential oils can enhance our feeling of well-being. Some essential oils, such as jasmine, are well liked by most people, whereas others (patchouli being a prime example) provoke a more extreme reaction, being loved by some but heartily disliked by others.

Kirlian photography can be used to reveal a person's electromagnetic field – the colours in this pair of hands are strong and vibrant, showing good health.

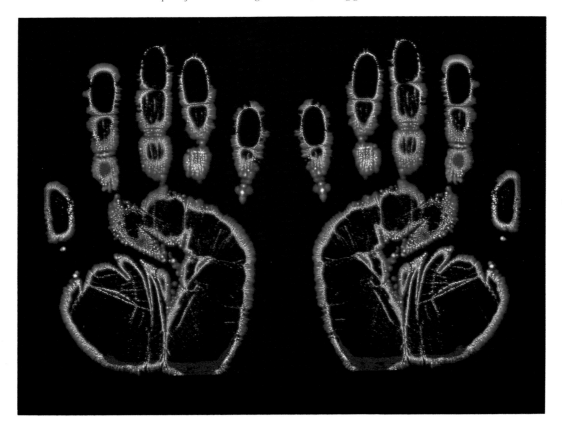

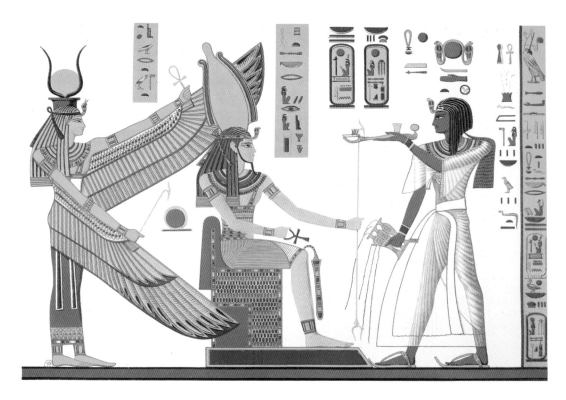

The Ancient Egyptians regarded fragrant oils as an essential part of worship. The man on the right approaches the two gods with an overflowing pot of aromatic oils in one hand, and an amschir (perfume-burner) held out in his left hand.

SPIRITUAL ESSENCES

Aromatic substances have been used for thousands of years. The Ancient Egyptians left particularly clear records in their murals and carvings showing how fragrant compounds were used a variety of purposes, including ritual, therapeutic and cosmetic. Other ancient civilizations also used fragrant substances; the oldest still for producing essential oils that has been found is from the Indus Valley of what is now Pakistan, and is 5000 years old. Thus, alongside other forms of plant medicine, such as herbalism, aromatherapy can be seen to be one of the most ancient forms of medicine.

To the ancients, there was no division between the sacred and the non-sacred. People's relationship with their gods was as important as their relationship with their neighbours, and if they became ill, the cause could be looked for on the spiritual as well as the physical plane. This means that medicines such as herbs and oils were chosen for their perceived spiritual activity as well as their physical properties. Aromatic substances were particularly important because as they possessed both a physical presence (for example the resin) and an invisible presence (the smell) they were used as a link between the seen and unseen, the spirit world and the world of form. This is one of the reasons why incense is such a universal substance of ritual: the smoke of the burning incense can be understood as carrying the fragrance and thereby prayers up to the gods.

This theme of aromatic substances being linked with the divine was developed by the alchemists of the Arabic world and then Europe. The practice of distillation was an important part of alchemy and various stages of the distillation processs were equated with stages of inner psychic transmutation. In the seventeenth century, the famous English herbalist Culpeper, himself drawing on much older sources, described the properties or 'virtues' of plants and designated a ruling planet or

astrological sign to many of them. Lavender and marjoram, for example, are described as under the dominion of Mercury, while pine is ruled by Mars. This link between a plant and a planet may still be used today by anyone with a knowledge of astrology to give an insight into the character of a plant or its essential oil.

Another way you can develop a greater understanding of the more profound character of an essential oil is to reflect or meditate on it. This process, described in depth in a book by Patricia Davis called *Subtle Aromatherapy*, is open to anyone who is able to let go of their everyday thoughts and tune into the symbolic level on which the oil is present. This is mainly the process by which the psychological profiles of the essential oils in this book have been developed. These are not necessarily complete and you may channel different or additional information about an oil as you begin to work with it. All aromatherapists develop their own relationship with the essential oils, and it is the marriage of the science of the oils with the human intuitive side that brings out the true healing and creative potential of aromatherapy.

Frankincense has been used as an aid to worship and prayers for millenia as a result of its unique combination of properties: calming and uplifting, while at the same time increasing energy and assisting concentration.

What are Essential Oils?

It is the essential oils within plants that give them their characteristic smell and flavour. When we smell the delightful fragrance of jasmine flowers in the early evening, open a cedarwood box and inhale its woody smell, or add the zest of a lemon to a drink, it is the essential oil that we are enjoying.

Any part of a plant may contain its essential oil – flowers, leaves, fruit, stems, wood, bark, seeds, resin, berries and roots. However, not all plants contain significant amounts of essential oils, and where this happens their purpose or function for those plants is not yet fully understood. It is thought that the oils' fragrance may attract or repel insects and other animals. Essential oils also have anti-viral and anti-fungal properties for the plant and can be understood as part of the plant's immune system. Other functions of essential oils within plants may be as plant 'hormones' and as an internal transport system (as with blood in animals).

Methods of extraction

An essential oil may be extracted from the plant material by one of four different methods. These four methods are described below.

DISTILLATION

Most of the essential oils that we use are produced by a process known as distillation. The plant material is placed in a container and boiling water or steam from a boiler is passed through the plant matter and then forced into an outlet pipe that carries away the vapours produced. The vapour passes through a pipe which runs through a jacket of flowing cold water (the condenser) and then drips into a second vessel that acts as a receiver for the condensed liquid.

During this process the boiling water or steam softens the tissues of the plant material and causes the release of the essential oil. This vapourizes and passes along with the steam through the vapour pipe, then both vapours condense to liquid in the area of the condenser. The mixture of liquid essential oil

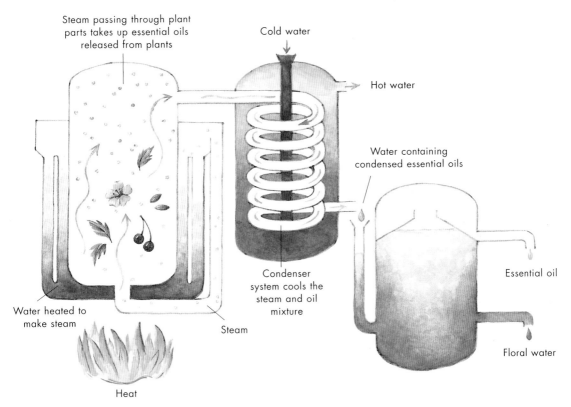

Steam passing through plant parts takes up essential oils released from plants

Cold water

Hot water

Water containing condensed essential oils

Condenser system cools the steam and oil mixture

Water heated to make steam

Steam

Essential oil

Floral water

Heat

Most essential oils are produced by distillation, the principle of which is shown in this diagram. Stills have been used to extract oils from plant matter for thousands of years.

and water then flows into the receiving vessel. Oil and water have different densities, so once they are in the receiving vessel they separate. The essential oil rises to the top, where it is drawn off, filtered and poured into containers ready for dispatch. Some essential oils are partially soluble in the distillation water, and in these cases the water may be recovered to use as a 'flower water' or distillate; rosewater or orangeflower water are obtained in this way.

Some essential oils are contained within hard, dense plant tissues, and this material has to be broken up or powdered before the essential oil can be released during distillation. Cedarwood, for example, is distilled from wood chips and sawdust collected from the sawmills where the wood has been cut for timber.

Stills used for essential oil production may be relatively small, such as those moved around the lavender fields in France on a trailer, or massive commercial machinery housed in large industrial buildings. Some ancient stills were made of terracotta; modern stills are usually stainless steel.

EXPRESSION

Citrus oils are obtained from oil glands found in the outer rind of the fruit and are generally not distilled but expressed. Expression used to be carried out by hand, rasping the peel against an abrasive surface and collecting the resulting liquid. Modern methods of expression vary from crushing the entire fruit, with subsequent separation of the oil from the peel and juice, to machine abrasion of the outer rind. Examples of essential oils that are usually produced by expression include sweet orange, bergamot, grapefruit and lemon; lime oil is usually distilled as this produces a finer product.

Most citrus oils, including orange oil, are obtained through expressing the peel.

ABSOLUTES

The essential oil found in jasmine flowers is too delicate to be produced by distillation; the heat tends to destroy the odour. In the past, a process known as enfleurage was used to extract the fragrance from flowers such as jasmine. This entailed placing the freshly picked flowers on to wooden-framed glass plates (chassis), upon which a layer of specially prepared fat had been spread. The chassis were stacked up overnight until the fat became saturated with the essential oil from the flowers.

Enfleurage was an extremely labour-intensive process, but became a well-known industry in the Grasse region of France. The fragrant enfleurage fat, known as pommade, was treated by extraction with alcohol to produce an absolute.

These days, most absolutes are not produced by such a romantic or craft-based method as enfleurage, but are made by solvent extraction. In this process the plant material is placed in a container with a volatile solvent, usually hexane. Blades are fitted to the inside of the drum and the contents are thoroughly mixed so that the solvent penetrates the plant tissue. The solvent will dissolve out the essential oil and also waxes, chlorophyll and any resinous matter. The extract is then placed in another vessel for the solvent recovery stage. The vessel is gently heated until the highly volatile solvent vapourizes off, leaving a residue known as the concrète or resinoid. In the final stage of production, the concrète is subjected to pure alcohol which separates the absolute from the residual wax. The alcohol solvent is then recovered, and the finished absolute is packed ready for dispatch.

Rose is most usually available as an absolute because of its high cost. While it is possible to produce rose oil by steam distillation, the yield tends to be relatively low and the resulting essential oil very expensive indeed.

Jasmine oil is destroyed by strong heat, so distillation cannot be used for this plant. Instead, the oil is mostly obtained through solvent extraction.

NITROGEN EXTRACTION AND CARBON DIOXIDE EXTRACTION

These methods of extracting essential oils have the advantage of not using heat as in distillation (the process is instead carried out under very high pressure), and not needing solvents other than the gas. It may be that we will see an increasing use of essential oils produced by gas extraction as we become more familiar and confident with them.

THE CHEMISTRY OF ESSENTIAL OILS

A single essential oil will usually be made up of hundreds of different chemical components. Each individual component will bring its own set of properties to the oil, so the total result is a very complex substance. All the constituents of an essential oil are organic – that is, their molecular structures contain carbon.

The chemical components of a typical essential oil generally occur as a combination of major, minor and trace constituents. An example of a major constituent is menthol, which makes up about 40% of peppermint oil. Typically, the number of major constituents is relatively small; the number of minor constituents is larger and the number of trace elements very large. It is the presence and combinations of these constituents that give each essential oil its characteristic smell. Some are so strong-smelling that even if they are not a major constituent they will still contribute greatly to the smell of the oil. Citral, for example, occurs in lemon oil as a minor constituent, and yet because the major constituents of lemon oil are relatively weak, it is the 'lemony' citral that we experience when we smell the oil.

Trace constituents may be so minute in an essential oil that their presence is expressed as so many parts per million. Nevertheless, some trace constituents are detectable by the human nose, and may still impart an important therapeutic value to the oil. An example of this is the constituent thioterpineol, which is a trace component of grapefruit oil, and is one of the most powerful-smelling substances known.

The majority of essential oil components fall into two categories: hydrocarbons, or terpenes, and oxygenated compounds.

TERPENES

Terpenes are composed of hydrogen and carbon atoms only, and are based on the chemical building block known as an isoprene unit. One important feature of terpene molecules is that they rapidly combine with oxygen from the air. This process starts off a chain reaction known as oxidation which unfortunately alters the odour and therapeutic properties of the affected essential oil for the worse. What this means is that essential oils rich in terpenes will oxidize and deteriorate in a short space of time. Lemon is an example of an essential oil rich in terpenes which will spoil quickly once exposed to air; the shelf life of lemon oil, once opened, is only about six to twelve months.

Essential oil of lemon contains only a small amount of citral, but it is the citral that gives lemons their distinctive scent.

There are two families of terpenes: monoterpenes and sesquiterpenes. Monoterpenes are particularly prone to rapid oxidation, and tend to have a weak smell. They are very common in essential oils and are a major constituent of orange oil, for example. Sesquiterpenes are less widely found in essential oils but tend to impart a strong smell to an oil. They are less prone to rapid oxidation. An example of a sesquiterpene is caryophyllene, which has a pungent, dry, woody odour and is a major component of clove oil.

OXYGENATED COMPOUNDS

The oxygenated compounds of essential oils belong to a number of different chemical families. Important examples are: alcohols which are in fact a group of terpene derivatives (for example geraniol, found in geranium oil); phenols, which are frequently skin irritants (thymol, found in thyme); aldehydes, which are quite widely found in essential oils and also tend to be skin irritants (citral, in lemongrass); esters, which often have a strong fruity odour (linalyl acetate, in bergamot oil); lactones (bergapten, in bergamot oil); and ketones, which are stable compounds not readily metabolized by the body (camphor, in rosemary oil).

What most of the oxygenated compounds have in common is that they are less prone to oxidation than the monoterpenes, and they tend to have a relatively strong smell. It is primarily the odour of the oxygenated compounds, and to a lesser extent the sesquiterpenes, that gives an essential oil its smell. It is, of course, the combination and presence of all these terpenes and oxygenated compounds that impart the therapeutic and also at times hazardous properties to an essential oil.

QUALITY

It is because a single essential oil is composed of hundreds of constituents, and each of those may be interacting with any of the others, that it is so difficult to replicate an essential oil synthetically. A pure essential oil is like a fine musical symphony, composed of hundreds of individual notes, and yet only in combination pleasing to the senses and beneficial to a person. With modern technology, it is not hard to synthesize several of the major components of an essential oil such as jasmine and combine them so that the smell is somewhat similar, yet the overall effect and benefit to an individual is insignificant compared to pure jasmine. A plastic rose may remind us of the real thing, but its presence will always be disappointing compared to the look, the touch, the smell and the overall experience of a true rose.

Synthetic or 'nature identical' oils are produced because they are cheaper than pure essential oils and also because they are more consistent. The manufacture of essential oils was developed to supply the food industry with flavours and the perfume industry with fragrances. The flavour and fragrance

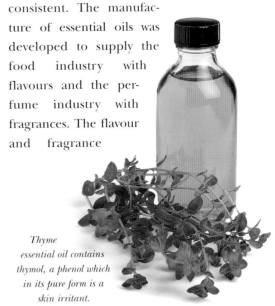

Thyme essential oil contains thymol, a phenol which in its pure form is a skin irritant.

market requirements are for a raw material that is cheap and exactly the same every year, not prone to variations as growing conditions change from harvest to harvest. It is only in recent years that aromatherapy has become popular and aromatherapists have begun to demand essential oils guaranteed to be pure and natural for their therapeutic use.

It is very difficult as an individual customer to determine that an essential oil from a supplier is totally pure and natural. Most 'adulterated' essential oils will not be an easily identified synthetic copy, but a blend of a true essential oil with an amount of a 'nature

Grapefruit oil contains traces of thioterpineol, one of the most powerful-smelling substances known.

identical' material added to increase the volume and thereby reduce the cost. A relatively more expensive essen-tial oil will be bulked out by adding a similar-smelling much cheaper oil, such as the addition of cheaper cananga oil to more

expensive ylang ylang. Finally, some essential oils may already be diluted by the addition of a base oil, such as almond. This may be promoted by some companies as a method of offering some of the very expensive oils, such as rose, at a more affordable price.

The best guarantee of quality is to buy your essential oils from a supplier who has a good reputation and a genuine interest in the therapeutic properties of its range. Back-up material that should be available on request could include the country of origin of a particular oil, the variety (Latin name), batch number and year of production.

Companies supplying essential oils will take certain measures to ensure the quality of their oils. They can visit the producers on a regular basis, which is practical for some oils such as the European ones, but less so for those from, say, Madagascar. There are also quality tests which are becoming increasingly accurate in determining the purity of an essential oil. Simple tests include visual inspection, odour, specific gravity and refractive index. Larger companies will also carry out gas liquid chromatography (GLC) on all batches of essential oil. During a GLC, the vapour of a small amount of essential oil is separated out into its individual components. The results of this separation are recorded by the instrument as a series of peaks on a sheet of paper, with each peak corresponding to a single constituent. The GLC analysis taken from a new batch of oil, say lavender oil, will then be compared against a standard lavender oil analysis to check that the number and ratio of constituents is acceptable.

No amount of testing, including even GLC analysis, is a total guarantee of purity, but the more steps that a company takes to establish quality, the more likely it is that a pure and natural essential oil is being offered.

Pesticides and herbicides are frequent contaminants of essential oils. If used on the crop during its cultivation, they will be carried through the expression or distillation process. This is a huge problem that has developed out of modern agricultural practices. The amount of pesticide and herbicide residue in essential oils is about the same as that considered acceptable in foods, but fortunately most pesticides and herbicides are not as readily absorbed into the system through human skin, when applying a massage oil for example, as they are when eating contaminated food.

One positive step that can be taken here is to buy essential oils that are wild-crafted or organically produced. Some companies do supply a range of essential oils that are certified as organically produced by the Soil Association in the UK, or other organic organization of the country of production. Buying these oils means not only that you are getting an essential oil uncontaminated by synthetic fertilizers and biocides, but you are also supporting the move towards sustainable agriculture and healthier produce.

Storage

The factors that will cause an essential oil to deteriorate are light, heat and oxygen. The best essential oil for therapeutic purposes is the freshest one. Sunlight is particularly damaging, and is capable of catalysing the reactions that cause deteriotation. For this reason, essential oils should be stored in coloured glass bottles and preferably kept in the dark. Do not keep essential oils, or even made-up massage oils, in plastic containers as there tends to be a chemical reaction between the plastic and certain essential oil components that will spoil the odour and therapeutic properties of the oil.

Essential oils should be stored in a cool place. An unheated room is adequate for many oils, but oils rich in terpenes, such as citrus and pine, are particularly prone to deterioration through heat and should be stored in the refrigerator. All essential oils will keep for longer in the refrigerator, although some of the resinous oils, such as cedarwood, and the absolutes will tend to become rather viscous at lower than room temperature and will have to be removed from the refrigerator for a while before they can be poured. If there are young children in the house, a childproof lock should be attached to the door of the refrigerator.

It is better to buy small quantities of essential oils regularly, but if you wish to buy a larger quantity it is advisable to pour it into a number of small bottles (about 10 ml) for storage. This is because each time a bottle is opened more oxygen enters the bottle, accelerating the process of oxidation.

The shelf life will vary from oil to oil and according to the conditions under which it is stored. The following guidelines apply to essential oils that are stored under cool, dark conditions: essential oils rich in terpenes, such as citrus oils, pine and rosemary, will deteriorate most quickly and should be used within 6–12 months of purchase; cedarwood, patchouli, sandalwood, vetiver and other resinous essential oils will keep for up to 3 years; and most other essential oils should be used within 2 years.

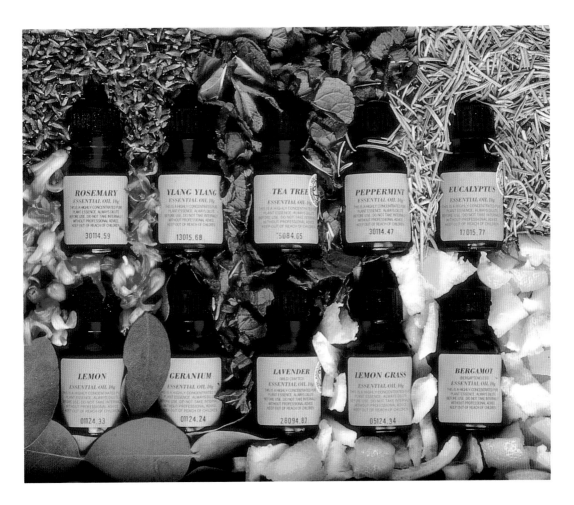

Essential oils need to be stored in dark bottles. Keep the oils in small quantities for storage, so that the oils are exposed to the air less than if they were in large bottles. This will restrict the process of oxidation, helping to preserve the oils.

Safety

When properly diluted and used with common sense, essential oils are safe, pleasurable and therapeutic and can greatly enhance a healthy lifestyle. They are, however, extremely concentrated plant essences and need to be treated with respect. Never apply any oils except those you know to be totally non-toxic and non-irritant directly to the skin without diluting first as detailed in this book. Do not take essential oils internally without supervision from an experienced and qualified practitioner. Do learn about the individual oils and use them cautiously at first and then with more confidence as your experience and knowledge grow.

If you have sensitive skin, do a patch test before using a new oil. Apply the diluted oil to a small patch of skin on the inner wrist or elbow and wait for an hour to check that no irritation or redness develops before using the oil more widely. If any adverse reaction at all develops after using a particular essential oil, discontinue its use immediately. It is possible to develop a sensitivity to any substance, including an essential oil, even after you have used it many times before.

The following guidelines will help you to use the oils discussed in this book safely, but if you have a professional interest in aromatherapy I would recommend that you read *Essential Oil Safety* by Robert Tisserand and Tony Balacs, a useful and detailed book.

ACCIDENTS WITH ESSENTIAL OILS

If you accidentally spill a neat essential oil on your skin, or develop an allergic reaction to an oil, splash plenty of cold water over the area and continue applying cold water for at least 20 minutes. If any irritation remains, consult your health practitioner. If any essential oil gets into the eyes, splash copiously with cold water and get urgent medical help if any redness or irritation persists. Several essential oils that are safe to use externally are toxic if

ESSENTIAL OILS TO AVOID

The following essential oils should not be used by anyone. Many are not available as they are already on government 'Poisons Lists' and are not allowed to be sold:

Armoise, bitter almond, boldo, buchu, cade, calamus, camphor (brown and yellow), cassia, cinnamon bark, costus, elecampane, exotic basil (high estragole), fig leaf, ho leaf (camphor and saffrol chemotypes), horseradish, hyssop, mustard, pennyroyal, sage (Dalmation), sassafras, tansy, tarragon, thuja, verbena, wintergreen, wormseed, wormwood.

taken internally, for example eucalyptus. If poisoning from an essential oil is suspected, telephone a general practitioner or go to the hospital accident and emergency department. If there are any serious signs of poisoning, such as seizures or unconsciousness, or a young child has ingested some essential oil, call the emergency services.

BABIES AND CHILDREN

Infants are much more sensitive than adults to the properties of essential oils and so the quantities used should always be only a quarter of the amounts used for adults. Young babies have particularly sensitive skin and should not be subjected to any oils that can be possible irritants.

If you have children in your house you should take steps to prevent them from getting hold of essential oils, just as you would with any medicine. Ensure that all your bottles have dropper inserts securely fitted. Keep all essential oils in a cupboard out of the reach of children, or, if you keep them in the refrigerator, fit a childproof catch to the door.

0–6 months: The only oils that should be used at this stage are lavender and Roman chamomile. Add 1 drop of essential oil to 10 ml/2 tsp of sweet almond oil or jojoba oil for a massage, or use in a room fragrancer.

6–12 months: Use only aniseed, chamomile and Roman chamomile, lavender, mandarin, neroli and rose.

1–6 years: Use only aniseed, chamomile and Roman chamomile, coriander, lavender, mandarin, neroli, orange, palmarosa, rose, rosewood and tea tree.

7–12 years: Use essential oils as indicated in this book, but avoid basil. Quarter the dosage given for adults of all the oils.

PREGNANCY

Used at normal aromatherapy dilutions, most essential oils are perfectly safe to use during pregnancy and can be very helpful in dealing with any problems or discomforts that arise during this time. It used to be considered that many oils that are unsafe to use internally during pregnancy because they might stimulate menstruation (emmenagogues) were also unsafe to use externally. There is no evidence to support this and essential oils such as juniper, marjoram, rose and rosemary are safe to use externally during pregnancy at normal aromatherapy dilutions. The exception is sage oil, which should be avoided during pregnancy.

HIGH BLOOD PRESSURE

Some aromatherapists have suggested that some of the more stimulating essential oils, such as rosemary, should be avoided by people with high blood pressure. There is in fact no evidence to support this view. The only exception is for people who suffer from cardiac fibrillation, who should avoid peppermint oil.

Using Essential Oils

Essential oils have been used for cosmetic, perfumery and therapeutic purposes for thousands of years. They are an invaluable part of the food and flavouring industry and in more recent years have also been incorporated into a wide range of commercial household and pharmaceutical products. Peppermint oil, for example, is used in confectionery, drinks, washing-up liquid, air fresheners, toothpaste, shaving foam and indigestion tablets, to name but a few of the commodities in which it appears.

Aromatherapy as we know it today has been developed during this century, originally by a small number of researchers investigating the antiseptic properties of essential oils. These became particularly important during the First World War, when certain oils were widely used to treat trench foot and infected wounds. One of these researchers was the Frenchman René-Maurice Gattefossé, who became the first person to use the word 'aromatherapie'.

In the 1960s aromatherapy was introduced to Britain by a remarkable woman called Marguerite Maury. In France,

Maury developed a system of aromatherapy that utilized both the medicinal properties of essential oils and their ability to rejuvenate the skin and maintain youth. She then set up a clinic in England and began to teach her system to beauty therapists, who became the first generation of holistic aromatherapists in Europe.

One of the areas that aromatherapists have researched is how essential oils are absorbed into the body. Gattefossé discovered that it takes between 30 minutes and 12 hours for an essential oil to be absorbed into the various systems of the body after massaging on to the skin. Since then, tests have shown that essential oil molecules can be detected in urine an hour after rubbing the oil on to the back of the hand. A simple test that you can do yourself is to rub a sliced garlic clove on to the soles of a friend's foot; after about 30 minutes you will be able to smell the essential oil from the garlic on his or her breath.

Peppermint essential oil is used in a wide variety of commercial products, including drinks, indigestion tablets and toothpaste.

How oils enter the body

The quickest way of drawing an essential oil into the system is by inhalation through the nose. When an odorous vapour is inhaled (for example, by wafting a tissue with a few drops of eucalyptus oil on it under the nose) the vapour is warmed and mixed with water vapour from the mucous membrane in the nasal cavity. The vapour molecules are then diffused over hundreds of microscopic hairs called cilia which are located in the olfactory organ at the root of the nose. Particular cilia are stimulated by different odours and a nervous impulse is sent to the adjacent olfactory bulb and then straight to the hypothalamus and limbic portions of the brain. (This part of the brain is the seat of the emotions, which explains why certain smells affect our moods and stir our memories so profoundly.) Neurochemicals are then released which are passed on, via the nervous system, to the rest of the body.

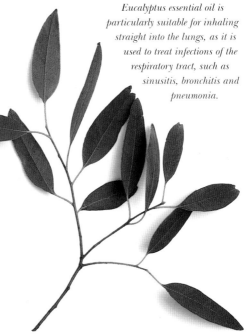

Eucalyptus essential oil is particularly suitable for inhaling straight into the lungs, as it is used to treat infections of the respiratory tract, such as sinusitis, bronchitis and pneumonia.

Inhaled essential oils will also pass into the lungs via the trachea and the bronchi, and from there into the bronchioles and eventually to the microscopic alveoli, where gaseous exchange with the blood takes place. The circulatory system will then transport them around the rest of the body.

There are a number of ways in which you can apply essential oils to the skin. Essential oil molecules are minute and penetrate the skin by diffusing through the hair follicles and sweat glands. They also permeate between the skin cells by combining with the skin's lipids (fats) and thereby enter the dermis (the layer of skin beneath the epidermis). Once in the dermis they can enter the blood capillaries and lymph vessels, which then transport them around the rest of the body by the circulatory systems.

ABSORBING OILS THROUGH THE SKIN

Exactly how much of an essential oil applied to the skin is absorbed into the body is variable and depends on the particular oil being used, the type of carrier (whether oil or water) and on the temperature of the surrounding air and of the oil itself (warmth increases absorption).

One of the main functions of the skin is as an organ of protection for the body, and this makes it particularly suitable as a route for the intake of essential oils, because the skin contains enzymes that can break down or inactivate several of the more potentially toxic constituents of the oils. There is no such protective system when the oils are taken internally. The layers of the skin also act as a kind of reservoir for essential oils, which are 'time-released' into the circulatory system. This means that essential oils are released into the body more slowly via the skin than if they are taken internally.

TAKING OILS INTERNALLY

When taken internally, essential oils are absorbed through the gastrointestinal tract straight into the bloodstream and thence to the liver. Oral administration of essential oils means that the entire dose is released into the system at once. One result of this is that any toxicity is most hazardous if the oil is taken internally; there is also the risk of irritation and damage to the lining of the gastro-intestinal tract.

Although taking essential oils internally can be extremely effective in the treatment of certain diseases, they should only be used in this way if prescribed by qualified medical practitioners who are specifically trained in the oral administration of essential oils. The same is true for rectal administration and vaginal douches: the mucous membranes of these areas are so delicate that these methods of application should be supervised by experienced practitioners. (See also information on Safety on pages 28–9, and safety notes on individual oils.)

HOW TO APPLY ESSENTIAL OILS

Most essential oils should be diluted before applying them to the skin, though there are a few exceptions. Lavender, jasmine, neroli, sandalwood and rose can generally be used neat as a perfume, and some wonderful blends can be made using these oils. Lavender and tea tree can be applied neat as a remedy for insect bites, minor burns and so forth or to disinfect wounds.

Methods of Application

MASSAGE

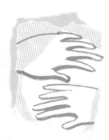

Massage is one of the most popular ways of using essential oils and is the method favoured by professional aromatherapists. With an aromatherapy massage you get the benefit of the massage itself as well as the benefits of the essential oils. Massaging a blended oil into your own skin can be very beneficial too, and may easily be made part of a daily skin and health care routine.

To create a massage oil you will need to dilute the essential oils into a base or carrier oil (see page 128). A therapeutic massage oil usually contains 1–3% of essential oil to base oil. For practical purposes, it is assumed that there are just over 20 drops of essential oil to 1 ml. This means that to 100 ml/3½ fl oz/scant ½ cup of base oil, 20–60 drops of essential oil (or of combined essential oils) are added. If you make up enough massage oil to last for several applications, store it in a dark-coloured glass bottle and use it within 6–12 months. You may substitute a lotion base for the carrier oil if you prefer.

To make enough blended oil for just one massage, pour approximately 10 ml/ 2 tsp of base oil on to a saucer and add 4–6 drops in total of your chosen essential oil or combination of oils.

There are many massage courses available that will help you to learn the different techniques of massage. If you practise first on yourself, and then on a friend or partner, you will become more confident about using your hands, and discovering what is pleasurable and beneficial. It is important for the recipient to feel warm and comfortable during a massage, and you should ensure that your hands are warm before touching the skin. Concentrate on any areas that are causing discomfort – for example, rub the oil into the abdomen to relieve period pains or colic. Covering the skin with a towel or cloth after the massage helps to keep the recipient warm and also encourages absorption of the essential oils.

For some suggested massage blends, see page 133–7.

BATHS

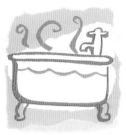

Adding essential oils to the bath is a wonderfully pleasurable and very popular way of using them. The warmth of the water encourages relaxation and also enables the essential oils to penetrate the skin. The oils should only be added to the water once the bath has been run, as the heat will encourage their evaporation.

Only the essential oils that are absolutely non-irritant, such as Roman chamomile and lavender, should be added direct to the bath; add 4–6 drops of essential oil or oils and swirl the water around before stepping in. Most essential oils should be pre-diluted in a carrier because they will not fully disperse in the water and their molecules may well come into direct contact with the skin and mucous membranes. Suitable pre-diluting substances include base oils, specially prepared bath oil bases which have a dispersant added, and full-fat milk. To prepare a bath using a carrier, mix 4–6 drops of essential oil in an eggcupful of milk or 10 ml/2 tsp of base oil, add the mixture to the bath and swirl the water before stepping in.

Sitz baths A sitz bath is an excellent way of treating haemorrhoids, thrush, pruritis, stitches following childbirth, and so on. Half-fill a large bowl or small bath with warm water. Use the same method of dilution as for baths, and sit in the water for 10 minutes. Adding tea tree oil to a sitz bath is the classic treatment for thrush.

Handbaths and footbaths Handbaths can be a part of a skin care routine, a way of treating pain and swelling of the hand joints, or just a very quick and easy way to create a general reviving effect. Footbaths are excellent for treating problems such as athlete's foot, for alleviating foot pain and swelling, and for helping to relieve discomfort in other parts of the body through the reflexology points found on the foot. To make a hand- or footbath add 4–6 drops of essential oil to a washing-up bowl full of hot water. Place your hands or feet in the bowl and soak for 10 minutes. A lavender footbath after a day on your feet is one of the most blissful experiences imaginable!

COMPRESSES

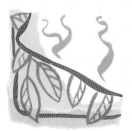

A hot compress is an effective way of treating many local complaints, such as skin infections, including abscesses and boils, and muscular or joint problems, including arthritis, rheumatism, sprains, strains, backache and so on.

To make a hot compress, pour hot water into a bowl and then add the essential oil. When treating a small area, such as a single boil, an eggcupful of hot water and 2 drops of essential oil will suffice; for a larger area, use a large bowl of water and 6–8 drops of essential oil. Place a cotton cloth in the water, ensuring that the cloth comes into contact with the essential oils on the surface, squeeze out the excess water from the cloth and then immediately put it on the painful or infected area. Keep the area warm by wrapping it in clingfilm (plastic wrap) and then wrap a towel around the clingfilm (plastic wrap). This process may be repeated after 20 minutes; keep the compress in place for about 1 hour. A hot compress made with ginger essential oil combined with cypress, juniper, pine and lavender is wonderfully warming and relieving for rheumatism or arthritis.

A cold compress may be preferred for certain types of headache and also if the area already feels over hot and inflamed. To make a cold compress, pour cold water into a bowl and add some ice cubes. Put 4–6 drops of essential oil into the water and then dip in the cotton cloth, wring it out and place it over the affected part. An ice pack (or a pack of frozen vegetables) can then be placed over the cloth to keep the area cold.

ROOM SPRAYS

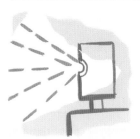

BURNERS AND VAPOURIZERS

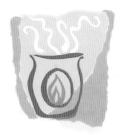

Room sprays can be used to disinfect and deodorize a room, repel insects and fumigate a sickroom. To make a room spray, half-fill a plant spray with water, add 40–60 drops of essential oils of your choice, shake well then spray liberally around the room.

Essential oils with good antiseptic properties, such as cedarwood, eucalyptus, lavender and tea tree, are ideal to use in sprays to fumigate rooms, while lemon, lemongrass and citronella can be used in a spray to repel insects. Most essential oil can be used to fragrance a room, but the citrus oils are particularly refreshing.

These can be used to deodorize or fumigate a room, or simply to create a special atmosphere. If you sit near to the burner or vapourizer it can also be a useful way of inhaling the vapours and benefiting from the therapeutic properties of the oil. Essential oil burners that use either a candle or electric power to heat the oils are on sale; put a little warm water on to the 'hot plate' and then add a few drops of essential oil.

Vapourizers are especially good for a child's room as they have a fan inside that disperses the vapour rather than using a source of heat.

INHALATIONS

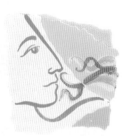

A steam inhalation is an excellent way of treating coughs, colds and sore throats and of deep-cleansing the skin. Put very hot water into a bowl and add 3–4 drops of essential oil. Then lean over the bowl, place a large towel over your head and the bowl to create a tent to contain the steam, and inhale the vapours.

Steam inhalations should be used with caution by people with epilepsy or asthma as they can be rather overpowering.

A quick and easy method of inhalation is to add 2–3 drops of essential oil to a tissue, and hold this near to the nose every few moments to inhale the vapours.

SAUNAS

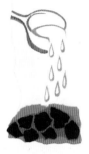

Essential oils make a wonderful addition to saunas. Simply add 20–40 drops of an essential oil or oils to the pitcher of water that is used to splash the coals during a sauna.

Cypress, eucalyptus and pine essential oils are particularly appropriate for use in the sauna.

GARGLES AND MOUTHWASHES

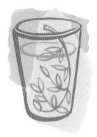

Gargles are a good way to treat sore throats and hoarseness, whether these have arisen from straining the voice or from a cold or infection. They can also be extremely effective in treating thrush, mouth ulcers and gum disease. Apart from totally non-irritant and non-toxic oils such as lavender and Roman chamomile, the oils must be diluted in a carrier before gargling. Add 2–3 drops of essential oil to 5 ml/1 tsp strong alcohol (vodka is ideal) and add this to an eggcupful of water. A mouthwash is made by adding the same amounts of alcohol and oil to warm water.

To make up a larger amount of mixture, put 50 ml/2 fl oz/¼ cup of vodka into a bottle and add 30–40 drops of essential oil. Add 5 ml/1 tsp of this mixture to warm water to use as your mouthwash or gargle.

COOKING

Essential oils have been used as flavourings for foods and drinks for many years. The main thing to remember is that they are very concentrated and so only 1–2 drops should be used per dish or the result will be too overpowering – and possibly toxic. The essential oil should be added to the liquid part of a recipe and mixed thoroughly to ensure that it is dispersed throughout the dish.

One of the simplest ways to start is to add 1–2 drops of fennel or lemon essential oil to mayonnaise as an accompaniment to fish. One or two drops of orange or neroli oil is delicious in home-made chocolates, and 1 drop of lime or spearmint oil will transform avocado soup.

PERFUMES

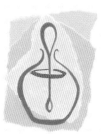

There are several essential oils that will not irritate the skin and may be worn undiluted as perfumes, including neroli, lavender, jasmine, sandalwood and rose. Simply apply a drop of the oil to the pulse points as you would any perfume. These oils may also be blended to create an individual fragrance, such as the classic combination of jasmine, rose and sandalwood, which is known as angel oil.

Colognes may also be created by adding a combination of essential oils to vodka as a fragrance base. Add up to 18 drops of combined essential oils to 30 ml/2 tbsp vodka and store in a glass perfume bottle.

HOW TO USE THE SYMBOLS

The symbols described here appear throughout the following pages as a quick reference to the way in which the individual essential oils may be used. Once you have become familiar with the symbols, you will find it easy to flick through the Oils section to find the appropriate oils for your needs. For example, if you would like to use an oil to fragrance a room, or for a massage blend, or as a flavouring in food, simply look through the oils section to find which oils carry the appropriate symbols, and decide which of those oils is best suited to your particular needs.

The Oils

This section contains profiles of the 42 main essential oils used in aromatherapy. Each profile contains information on the origin of the essential oil and its traditional or historical uses, with the method of extraction and a description of the oil. Each essential oil is different, with its own characteristic combination of properties, both therapeutic and psychological. These are described, with details of how the oil may be used to treat ailments or simply to improve overall health and well-being. Important information about safety and quick-reference symbols indicating use are also included.

Rosewood

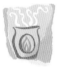

Aniba rosaeodora

Also known as: Bois de rose

Family: Lauraceae

ORIGIN

The rosewood tree is a medium-sized evergreen from the Amazon basin. The timber is used for making carvings and furniture. Sadly, rosewood is among the trees that are being felled in the destruction of the South American rainforests, and most of the essential oil has been produced from timber resulting from these clearances. For this reason many companies have stopped selling it unless they can establish that the supply is from sustainably managed plantations. Distillation is mainly carried out in Brazil and Peru.

THERAPEUTIC PROPERTIES

Rosewood is a balancing and gentle oil that acts as a mild tonic, pleasant to use in massage and bath oils and delightful in an essential oil burner. Because it is mild and non-toxic it is safe for children. It blends well with bergamot, cedarwood, clove, rose, frankincense, lemon, mandarin, sandalwood and ylang ylang.

Rosewood has a mild tonifying action on the nervous system and also has a balancing action, being both calming and uplifting. It can help to clear the head and aid concentration and is excellent for this when used in an essential oil burner. It can also help to relieve headaches, especially those associated with stress and tension, and is good for many other disorders that are related to stress.

This oil has aphrodisiac properties and is particularly appropriate in the treatment of frigidity. Use it as a massage or bath oil and also to fragrance and add a sensual atmosphere to the room.

As a gentle tonic for the immune and lymphatic systems, dilute rosewood in a base oil and massage over areas of enlarged or tender lymph glands. It may also be used in steam inhalations

METHOD OF EXTRACTION

Rosewood essential oil is steam- or water-distilled from chipped wood. It used to be a major source of the component linalool, widely used in perfumery, although in recent years most linalool has been synthetically produced.

to treat lingering viral infections, especially those associated with depression. A mild expectorant, it will relieve a dry, irritating cough – use in a steam inhalation or burn in the room.

Rosewood has a tonifying action on the digestive system and is mildly aperient. It may be massaged over the abdomen to relieve constipation. It will also help to relieve headaches associated with nausea or constipation.

The anti-inflammatory and soothing properties of rosewood make it helpful in skin care, relieving hot, dry and inflamed skin conditions. It also has regenerative properties and can be used to treat scarring, tired skin and wrinkles.

Psychological profile

Rosewood is a profoundly healing oil that can be used in times of crisis. It helps to steady the nerves and keep you calm while at the same time lifting the spirits and imparting a feeling of well-being. It is particularly suitable for children going through a time of transition.

DESCRIPTION

A colourless or pale yellow liquid, rosewood oil has a very pleasant sweet, woody and floral odour.

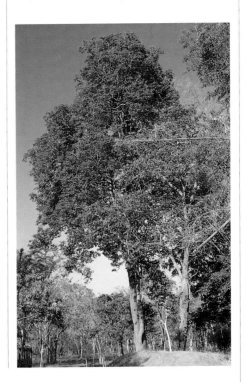

MOST COMMON USES

Stress • Aphrodisiac
Lymphatic tonic • Skin care

Safety data

Non-toxic • Non-irritant • Non-sensitizing

Frankincense

Boswellia thurifera, syn. B. carteri

Also known as: Olibanum

Family: Burseraceae

ORIGIN

Frankincense has been in constant demand since the time of the Ancient Egyptians, who used it in skin care preparations. It also has a tradition of use as incense in China, India and the West. Frankincense trees grow wild in North Africa, but the oil is mainly distilled from the resin in Europe.

THERAPEUTIC PROPERTIES

Frankincense is a tonifying oil with anti-inflammatory and astringent properties. It is a wonderful rejuvenating oil to use in massage and skin lotions, though its uplifting properties are best experienced by adding it to an essential oil burner; it may also be added to the bath. Frankincense blends particularly well with citrus oils, spice oils and basil, cedarwood, myrrh, neroli, pine, sandalwood and vetiver.

The main action of frankincense is on the nervous system, where it imparts a calming and uplifting effect while at the same time increasing energy. Its ability to assist concentration indicates its long history of use as an incense and an aid to meditation. It can also be helpful in treating anxiety and tension; a few drops of frankincense in an essential oil burner are very uplifting and beneficial if you are feeling stressed, tired or overwhelmed.

Its astringent and anti-inflammatory properties make frankincense useful in the treatment of all mucus conditions and other discharges, such as diarrhoea. It has a soothing effect on the mucous membranes and can be used for coughs, bronchitis and laryngitis – use it as a steam inhalation or in an essential oil burner. Frankincense is more cooling than cypress oil and a better expectorant when treating lung conditions, but is less effective in treating circulatory disorders.

The tonifying and rejuvenating properties of frankincense make it

METHOD OF EXTRACTION

The bark is incised so that the tree yields an oleo-gum resin which is collected after it solidifies into amber-coloured lumps the size of a pea. This resin is then steam-distilled to produce the essential oil.

DESCRIPTION

Frankincense oil has a sweet, spicy, resinous odour with a fresh, slightly camphoraceous top note. It is pale yellow or greenish in colour.

one of the most important oils for improving skin tone and treating ageing skin and wrinkles, as well as reducing scar tissue. It is also antiseptic and astringent and will help to close wounds and heal ulcers.

PSYCHOLOGICAL PROFILE

Frankincense is appropriate if you live at high speed and become overwhelmed by the responsibilities and material aspects of life without making time to establish a more considered and harmonious lifestyle. It is of benefit for people who have become cluttered in their atmosphere and who constantly wish they had the time for all those creative and spiritual pursuits they would like to do. Using frankincense will help you to reprioritize your life and to concentrate on those areas that will bring you greater satisfaction and happiness.

Lumps of gum resin

MOST COMMON USES

Meditation • Stress
Mucus conditions • Ageing skin

SAFETY DATA

Non-toxic • Non-irritant in dilution • Non-sensitizing

45

Ylang ylang

Cananga odorata

Family: Annonaceae

ORIGIN

Ylang ylang oil is produced from the flowers of a tall tree native to tropical Asia, especially Indonesia. Commercial production is mainly undertaken in Madagascar, the Comoro Islands off the coast of East Africa and the island of Réunion. The name means 'flower of flowers', and the flowers have been used in folk medicine in the Far East for thousands of years. In Indonesia they are spread on the beds of newly married couples on their wedding night, and in both Indonesia and the Philippines they are used in skin creams, often with a coconut oil base. In Victorian England the essential oil was an ingredient of the popular hair treatment macassar oil, which was thought to stimulate hair growth. Ylang ylang oil is a renowned base note found in many oriental and floral perfumes.

THERAPEUTIC PROPERTIES

Ylang ylang has a sedating and calming effect on the nervous system while at the same time creating a sense of relaxed well-being. It is useful for treating anxiety, depression, stress and tension and blends well with bergamot, cedarwood, clary sage, jasmine, lemon, rose, sandalwood and vetiver. It should always be well diluted as it can be rather overpowering, causing headaches or nausea – just a drop or two of ylang ylang in a saucerful of base oil is sufficient for massage.

This is an important oil in the treatment of high blood pressure. It will help to lower blood pressure and reduce tachycardia (abnormally rapid heart beat) and hyperpnoea (abnormally fast breathing). It has a soothing effect on palpitations

METHOD OF EXTRACTION

The oil is steam- or water-distilled from the freshly picked flowers of the tree. During the distillation process a number of different grades of oil are taken off. The first is known as ylang extra, and this is the most expensive and most desired by perfumers. There then follow three successive distillates known as grades I, II and III, the smell of the different grades becoming less and less complex and losing more of the subtle top notes.

associated with anxiety and panic. In treating circulatory disorders ylang ylang may be blended with other appropriate oils and used in massage and the bath, though the best results will be obtained by visiting an aromatherapist for a therapeutic massage and advice on lifestyle.

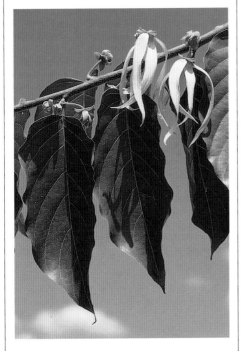

Ylang ylang has an excellent reputation as an aphrodisiac for both men and women, relaxing inhibitions and dispelling stress while at the same time being arousing. It can be effective as a sensual massage blend or as a room fragrancer.

DESCRIPTION

Ylang ylang oil is a pale yellow oily liquid with a very powerful floral, intensely sweet and exotic smell with a balsamic undertone.

Ylang ylang adds an exotic and luxurious fragrance to many skin care products as well as balancing the secretion of sebum. It is suitable for both dry and oily skin types and may be used in preparations to treat acne and problem skin.

PSYCHOLOGICAL PROFILE

Ylang ylang is most appropriate if you have pushed yourself to work hard and taken on many commitments until you are no longer in control of the stress in your life. You may have forgotten how to let go and enjoy yourself, having become tense, irritable and anxious, and may easily become flushed and panicky. Using ylang ylang will help you to relax and enable you to reprioritize your life so that you can begin to enjoy yourself again.

MOST COMMON USES

Anxiety • Aphrodisiac
High blood pressure

SAFETY DATA

Non-toxic • Non-irritant • Non-sensitizing

Cedarwood

Cedrus atlantica

Also known as: Atlas cedar

Family: Pinaceae

ORIGIN

Cedarwood has been valued since ancient times and the trees were used to build temples, including the temple of Solomon. The wood was prized for building because it is very hard and the natural oils present in the wood repel insects. Cedarwood essential oil was one of the earliest to be extracted, and was used by the Ancient Egyptians in cosmetics, perfumes and in the mummification process. The oil is now mainly produced in Morocco and France.

THERAPEUTIC PROPERTIES

Cedarwood is very warming as well as regenerating, tonifying, soothing and uplifting. The balancing nature of the last two properties makes it excellent in the treatment of nervous tension, chronic anxiety, depression and tiredness; it may be added to massage and bath oil blends and steam inhalations, and it is also a pleasant room fragrancer. Cedarwood blends particularly well with bergamot, cypress, frankincense, jasmine, juniper, myrrh, neroli, rosemary, sandalwood and vetiver.

Its regenerative properties make cedarwood useful in the treatment of chronic conditions such as arthritis – blend with other appropriate oils in a base oil and use for massage or as a compress. It is tonifying where there is weakness combined with excessive discharges, such as chronic diarrhoea or excessive urination, in which case it should be applied in a massage oil over the abdomen. Combined with sandalwood and used in the bath or as a douche, cedarwood may also be used to treat cystitis.

This oil will help to stimulate delayed periods, and its antiseptic properties also make it a good treatment for leucorrhoea, discharges and venereal infections. Add a few drops to the bath to bring relief to pruritis. In a therapeutic compress it will prevent putrefaction in wounds, ulcers including varicose ulcers, and any

METHOD OF EXTRACTION

The oil is steam-distilled from the wood and sawdust.

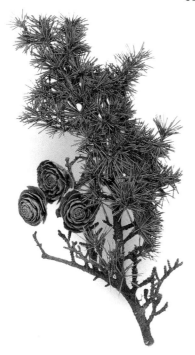

DESCRIPTION

Cedarwood oil may be yellow or amber and is quite viscous. It has a slightly sweet, oily-woody smell that becomes more woody as it dries out.

PSYCHOLOGICAL PROFILE

Cedarwood is appropriate if you have problems with self-identity or are prone to daydreams and fantasies which may become morbid or perverse. These will further increase the inability to integrate with the world and may even lead to mental degeneration. Cedarwood helps to give a stronger sense of identity and encourages interrelation with other people.

OTHER VARIETIES

There are two other varieties of cedarwood oil: Texas (*Juniperus ashei*) and Virginian (*Juniperus virginiana*). While they share similar therapeutic properties with Atlas cedarwood, they can cause skin irritation and sensitization and are best avoided for aromatherapy.

skin infection where the skin is degenerating.

Cedarwood has a beneficial effect on the mucous membranes, especially when there is excessive catarrh, and can be used to treat coughs and bronchitis. Use as a steam inhalation or burn in the room.

Its combination of antiseptic and astringent properties mean that cedarwood is a good treatment for oily skin and hair, acne, dandruff and scalp irritation, as well as fungal infections of the skin such as athlete's foot. It is also a parasiticide and may be combined with other oils to eliminate lice and scabies.

MOST COMMON USES

Nervous tension and anxiety • Acne
Dandruff • Coughs and bronchitis
Skin infections • Arthritis

SAFETY DATA

Non-toxic • Non-irritant in dilution • Non-sensitizing

Cinnamon

Cinnamomum zeylanicum

Family: Lauraceae

ORIGIN

The cinnamon tree is a native of east India and Indonesia. The inner bark of the young twigs, sold as cinnamon sticks, has been used in cooking and as a medicine for thousands of years. In herbal medicine cinnamon is used to treat colds and flu, digestive disorders and rheumatism.

THERAPEUTIC PROPERTIES

Cinnamon is a pungent and warming oil with stimulating and tonifying properties. It is useful for strengthening and tonifying the circulatory, respiratory and digestive systems and is restorative for weak, tired, cold people. It can irritate the skin and must be very well diluted in a base oil before application; do not use in dilutions of stronger than 0.5% and do a patch test on a small area of skin before using. Because cinnamon can irritate the mucous membranes it should not be added to general bath oils, though it may be used in foot baths. It should never be applied to the face. Cinnamon blends particularly well with clove, eucalyptus, frankincense, lemon, mandarin and orange.

Cinnamon will stimulate a sluggish digestion, especially when aggravated by cold food, and will strengthen peristalsis in people prone to constipation; its antispasmodic properties will help to relieve any kind of digestive spasm, such as colic. Combine it with marjoram and orange, dilute well in a base oil and massage over the abdomen.

As a general tonifier, cinnamon may be blended into a massage oil and massaged into the lower back. This will help to strengthen the adrenal glands and general vitality as well as aiding in the cure of impotence. To treat chills and poor circulation to the extremities, add a few drops of cinnamon to a teaspoon of base oil, put in a bowl of very warm water and use as a foot or hand bath.

METHOD OF EXTRACTION

For aromatherapy purposes the essential oil is steam-distilled from the leaves and young twigs. An essential oil is also distilled from the bark, but this is extremely irritant and should not be used for aromatherapy.

Cinnamon oil is a yellow or brownish-yellow liquid with a harsh, warm and spicy odour.

Cinnamon can be used to treat rheumatism, especially when the pain is aggravated in cold, damp weather. Try combining it with lemon and juniper in a base oil and gently massaging the area.

The strongly antiseptic properties of cinnamon make it good for treating colds and flu; it works very well in an essential oil burner or in a room spray to fumigate a room. Cinnamon is also a useful parasiticide, especially for treating lice and scabies. For the former, combine it with oils of eucalyptus, pine, rosemary and thyme and comb through the hair; for the latter, combine with bergamot and cedarwood and apply to the skin.

PSYCHOLOGICAL PROFILE

Cinnamon is appropriate if you have become disappointed with life and feel that you will not achieve your earlier hopes. You may feel that you have become something of an outsider or even cynical and depressed. Using cinnamon will help to rekindle your interest and enthusiasm for life.

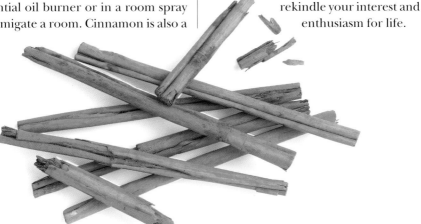

MOST COMMON USES

Sluggish digestion • Chills
Lice and scabies

SAFETY DATA

Non-toxic • Do not use in concentrations of more than 0.5%

Neroli

Citrus aurantium

Also known as: Orange blossom

Family: Rutaceae

ORIGIN

Neroli oil is produced from the flowers of the bitter orange tree, also known as the Seville orange. The tree is native to China, but has been cultivated for hundreds of years in the countries bordering the Mediterranean. Neroli oil is one of the classic perfume and eau de cologne ingredients. Orange-flower water is a renowned skin toner for dry and mature skin.

THERAPEUTIC PROPERTIES

Neroli is both calming and uplifting, although its effect in the long run is relaxing. It adds a wonderful fragrance to many massage and bath oil blends and combines particularly well with citrus oils, clary sage, jasmine, lavender and rosemary.

The main action of neroli is on the nervous system, and it is one of the most effective anti-depressant essential oils. People who feel exhausted, depressed, anxious and confused will benefit from neroli as it will aid sleep, promote relaxation and help to clear the mind and lift the spirits. It is also a useful first-aid treatment for shock and hysteria.

The relaxing effect of neroli also has an effect on heart problems arising from tension, including tachycardia and palpitations. Use it to create a relaxing bath and massage oil.

Neroli has antispasmodic properties which make it a good remedy for digestive cramps, especially those arising from a nervous origin. It may also be useful in treating diarrhoea, especially if it is of a chronic nature or stress-related. Try combining it with geranium and massaging it over the abdomen.

Another main area of neroli's actions is on the skin. The oil has a very low toxicity and its rejuvenating properties make it useful for treating dry, mature skin, wrinkles and broken capillaries. Applied during pregnancy, it will help to prevent stretch marks. It is said to stimulate the elimination of dead skin cells. It also has a deodorizing effect.

METHOD OF EXTRACTION

Neroli oil is water-distilled from the freshly picked flowers in May and October.

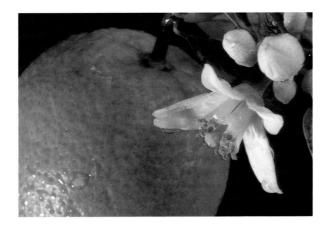

DESCRIPTION

A pale yellow liquid that becomes darker on ageing, neroli has an exquisite, floral, sweet smell which is powerful yet also light and refreshing.

PSYCHOLOGICAL PROFILE

To benefit most from neroli you will be a somewhat private person, slightly reserved and seemingly calm and cool; you may come across as a rather aloof and sophisticated type. However, while everything appears to be under control and to your liking, this may conceal considerable anxiety, worry and stress. Using neroli will allow you to relax and become more in touch with your heart, able to express your true emotions. This will lead to you feeling less remote from other people. Neroli will also help you to sleep better, relax more and participate in life more fully.

OTHER VARIETIES

Petitgrain essential oil is steam-distilled from the leaves and twigs of the same tree as neroli. It has a pleasant, fresh, floral and sweet smell with a herbaceous and slightly woody undertone. Like neroli, petitgrain has uplifting properties and the two can be combined. It is slightly more astringent than neroli and can be used to treat oily skin and acne.

MOST COMMON USES

Depression • Insomnia
Mature skin • Stretch marks

SAFETY DATA

Non-toxic • Non-irritant • Non-sensitizing

Orange

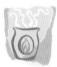

Citrus aurantium, syn. C. sinensis

Also known as: Sweet orange

Family: Rutaceae

ORIGIN

Orange trees are natives of the Far East, brought to Europe in the early sixteenth century and then taken on to the Americas by the Spanish and Portuguese. There are many varieties of orange tree, grown in different parts of the world. The essential oil has been produced in many countries for local use, for example in drinks. Today, most of the commercial production of orange oil is from Brazil, the USA and Cyprus.

THERAPEUTIC PROPERTIES

Orange oil is very pleasant to experience and also very safe because of its low toxicity and moderate effect. It may be used for children, who generally enjoy its fresh, sweet smell. A versatile oil, it is suitable for skin conditioners, massage oils, bath oils and room fragrancing, and blends particularly well with spice oils, other citrus oils, clary sage, geranium, lavender, myrrh, neroli and rosemary. This oil has a relaxing effect but is uplifting rather than overly sedating. Its pleasant fragrance makes it beneficial when treating stress, nervous tension and related headaches, especially those connected with the digestive system. In the latter instance, combine with chamomile for the best effect.

Orange has a moving action, good for the treatment of symptoms that arise from a sluggish or obstructed system, such as flatulence and constipation. Dilute in a base oil and massage over the abdomen.

The primary function of orange is on the liver and digestive system. It is one of the main liver unblockers, helpful when there is congestion of the liver or spleen; its action is very gentle and easily tolerated. It acts as a mild aperient, helping bowel movements by encouraging peristalsis, and will also alleviate colic. Orange combines well with fennel, aniseed and peppermint for prolonged digestive conditions.

METHOD OF EXTRACTION

The traditional method of obtaining orange oil was to hand-express it by rasping the peel, but most modern production is by machine expression.

DESCRIPTION

Orange oil is a pale orange-yellow colour with a sweet, fresh and fruity smell.

Orange oil has a general detoxifying and cleansing effect and will encourage the elimination of excess fluids and waste products from the system. Orange may be used as a massage or bath oil during a detoxifying programme and may be added to blends for the reduction of cellulite.

Due to its moderating and balancing effect, orange oil can be employed in the treatment of gastric fevers, colds and flu. Its tonifying and slightly astringent properties also indicate its appropriateness for oily or dull and tired skin.

PSYCHOLOGICAL PROFILE

Constitutionally, orange oil is suitable if you have trouble getting things done. You may have met many obstacles and become frustrated, eventually succumbing to laziness and finding it an effort to make any changes in your life. Bad habits of over-indulgence and avoidance of exercise may develop, and you will become overweight. Using orange oil will begin to accelerate the sluggish organic processes, and the tenor of your life will also begin to change as you become more optimistic and purposeful.

MOST COMMON USES

Slow digestion • Constipation
Overeating • Tension headaches
Tiredness

SAFETY DATA

Non-toxic • Non-phototoxic • Non-irritant in dilution • Sensitization rare

Bergamot

Citrus bergamia

Family: Rutaceae

ORIGIN

The bergamot orange is a species similar to the bitter orange. The most likely origin of the name is that it derived from Bergamo, in Lombardy, where the fruit was sold. Production of the essential oil started during the early eighteenth century in Italy, and since then bergamot oil has become one of the most important perfume materials. It is the main constituent of eau de cologne as well as being used in lotions, creams, perfumes, sweets and soaps. It is bergamot oil that gives Earl Grey tea its distinctive flavour.

THERAPEUTIC PROPERTIES

Bergamot is a cooling and refreshing oil. Its main action is on the nervous system, where it acts as a tonic, and is invigorating without being over-stimulating. It makes a pleasant, fragrant addition to many massage and bath oil blends, and combines particularly well with coriander, cypress, geranium, juniper, lavender, melissa, neroli, pine and rosemary.

Bergamot has a soothing effect, and is a good nerve tonic when tension makes you feel hot and sweaty. It is also useful for tension headaches. Its cooling and refreshing properties make it an oil that helps during times of stress and when you are feeling cross, irritable and overwrought. It blends well with melissa and rosemary to clear the mind.

Bergamot has carminative and anti-spasmodic properties which makes it useful for problems of the digestive system; especially where there is colic, painful wind and indigestion. The antiseptic properties of the oil can help in treating gastroenteritis and other gastric infections – massage it over the abdomen.

In Italy, bergamot is used for treating fevers as it is cooling and antiseptic. It has a special affinity for the mouth and throat and is traditionally employed in

METHOD OF EXTRACTION

Bergamot oil is produced by rasping the peel and collecting everything that is expressed. This is then clarified and filtered to become expressed oil of bergamot.

DESCRIPTION

Bergamot oil is a light, yellow or pale green liquid with an extremely rich, sweet, green and fruity smell.

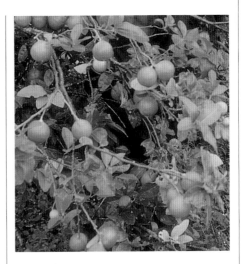

the treatment of sore throats, mouth ulcers and bad breath.

Bergamot oil alleviates genito-urinary infections where there is burning, heat and inflammation; use in the bath or as a douche. It is also widely used in the treatment of skin conditions for its antiseptic, healing and deodorizing properties and is particularly recommended in the treatment of acne, herpes, psoriasis and seborrhoea of the scalp.

This oil increases photosensitivity of the skin, which means the skin tans more readily. For this reason you must be careful not to apply bergamot to the skin before going out into the sun or you may burn very easily. It is possible to buy bergamot oil that has had the component bergaptene removed and this will not cause photosensitivity.

In first-aid, bergamot is used as an antiseptic in the treatment of wounds and ulcers. It will act as a parasiticide for eliminating scabies. It also makes a deodorizing and refreshing room spray.

PSYCHOLOGICAL PROFILE

Bergamot is an appropriate oil if you are the type of person who pursues goals in life with a determination to succeed at whatever cost. It is cooling and refreshing for the cross, critical, exacting person who begins to suffer from digestive and skin problems, and whose nerves become edgy and raw.

MOST COMMON USES

Tonic for the nervous system
Cooling and refreshing
Good for tension, stress and irritability
Indigestion • Cystitis
Wounds and ulcers

SAFETY DATA

Non-toxic • Non-sensitizing • Non-irritant
Use bergaptene-free bergamot, or do not use in concentrations of more than 0.4%
if applying to the skin within 12 hours of exposure to sunlight

Lemon

Citrus limonum

Family: Rutaceae

ORIGIN

The lemon tree is native to India but arrived in Europe with the Crusaders as long ago as the twelfth century. The essential oil has been commercially developed for its extensive use in the perfumery and flavouring industries.

THERAPEUTIC PROPERTIES

Lemon is primarily a refreshing, cleansing and tonifying oil, and is one of the most important bactericidal oils for any infection or putrefaction. It is a versatile oil to use in massage and bath oil blends, compresses, inhalations and room fragrancing. It blends well with nearly every other essential oil, and will provide a top note to 'lift' many fragrance blends.

Lemon is a tonic for the circulatory system and will improve a sluggish circulation and weak venous system which gives rise to chilblains or varicose veins. Its regular use is also said to reduce blood viscosity and help break down sclerotic deposits. It is a traditional remedy for the treatment of broken capillaries visible on the skin.

This oil has a tonifying and stimulatory action on the digestive system. It can be used to treat obesity and also debility, weakness and loss of appetite. It helps to stimulate the production of pancreatic and gastric juices, and its cleansing and detoxifying properties can be of benefit to congested liver conditions and cellulite.

The moving and antiseptic properties of lemon will alleviate many respiratory conditions by combating infection and helping to eliminate mucus – use in steam inhalations or a massage blend to rub on the chest to treat colds, flu, bronchitis and asthma. Lemon also helps to stimulate the production of white blood cells, thereby strengthening the immune response. It is a good preventative during epidemics of contagious disease – use it in an essential oil burner or a plant spray in the room.

The antiseptic and astringent properties of lemon are appropriate for greasy skin and also any skin

METHOD OF EXTRACTION

Lemon oil is machine-expressed from the ripe peel of the lemon.

DESCRIPTION

A transparent liquid with a fresh, sweet and green-citrus smell reminiscent of the ripe peel.

infection such as boils, acne, ulcers and eruptions. Make a lemon compress to treat boils and other eruptions.

Lemon's astringent and tonifying properties will combat wrinkles. It is also an anti-viral oil and, applied neat, will help to eliminate warts and verrucae.

Lemon can be used against scabies and other parasitic infestations. It has insect-repellent properties and will prevent insect bites from going septic. Spray it around the house to discourage household insects such as animal fleas and ants.

PSYCHOLOGICAL PROFILE

Lemon oil is appropriate if you feel you need an astringent and cleansing treatment. You may have greasy hair and skin and a sluggish digestion, and perhaps feel generally unclean. There may have been a period in your life when you have neglected to take full care of yourself, which generally stems from a lack of self-respect. You may have a tendency to body odour. Using lemon oil will help to tighten up your tissues and encourage you to feel healthier and cleaner and be more self-confident.

Lemons and limes

Lime

Lime (*Citrus auran-tifolia*) shares the refreshing and uplift-ing properties of lemon and blends well with all the citrus fruits. Lime oil is strongly phototoxic and should not be used in concentrations of more than 0.5% if going out into the sun within 12 hours of application.

MOST COMMON USES

Refreshing • Cleansing
Circulatory tonic • Greasy skin
Skin eruptions, boils
Insect repellent • Colds and flu

SAFETY DATA

Sensitization possible • Phototoxic – do not use in concentrations of more than 2% if going into sunlight within 12 hours of application

Grapefruit

Citrus paradisi

Family: Rutaceae

ORIGIN

The grapefruit is thought to have evolved from a citrus fruit known as shaddock, which is native to the Caribbean. Cultivation now occurs in the USA, South America, the Caribbean and Israel. There are many varieties of grapefruit, including ruby or pink grapefruit, which is also available as an essential oil. Grapefruits are rich in Vitamin C and are known as a cleansing and beneficial food.

THERAPEUTIC PROPERTIES

Grapefruit is a cooling and slightly astringent oil. It is a mild tonic and shares refreshing and detoxifying properties with other citrus oils. It makes a pleasant, refreshing addition to many bath and shower preparations and also massage blends. Grapefruit blends particularly well with other citrus oils, clove, cypress, ginger, lavender, neroli, palmarosa and rosemary.

The main action of grapefruit oil is on the liver, where it has a cooling and detoxifying effect. It can calm symptoms of irritability, anger and overheating, and is a wonderful morning pick-me-up to use in a shower gel or bath oil following a hangover, late night or overindulgence.

Grapefruit is a mild aperient and will encourage peristalsis and thus relieve constipation. It is one of the main essential oils used in the treatment of obesity. It can help to reduce the appetite and stimulate the rate of metabolism of fats.

It has a generally detoxifying effect on the body and can help with lymphatic cleansing and reducing cellulite. Grapefruit is excellent to use during a detoxifying programme. Use as a massage oil, or combine with Dead Sea Salts and add to the bath.

It also has a beneficial action on the respiratory system, and is good for treating colds and flu with hot, feverish symptoms. It may be combined with other appropriate oils such as eucalyptus or pine and used in a steam inhalation.

METHOD OF EXTRACTION

Grapefruit oil is machine-expressed from the peel of the ripe fruit.

DESCRIPTION

Grapefruit has a fresh, sweet, citrus smell, similar to sweet orange. The colour may be yellow, pale green or pale orange. As with other citrus oils, grapefruit oxidizes quickly and the odour and therapeutic properties will deteriorate after 6–12 months.

PSYCHOLOGICAL PROFILE

Grapefruit is appropriate if you are very self-conscious and unhappy about your appearance. You may put on weight easily, have problem skin or simply get embarrassed easily. You may also have a tendency to feel ashamed and that you are less worthy than other people. Using grapefruit will help to improve your sense of self-worth and help you to become more empowered and positive about yourself and what you can do with your life.

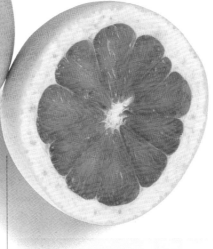

On the skin, grapefruit has cleansing, antiseptic, cooling and slightly astringent properties; it is helpful for oily skin, open pores and acne. Use in a lotion or as a facial steam. It will also help to tone and tighten loose skin, for example, after losing weight.

MOST COMMON USES

Detoxifying • Constipation
Cellulite • Hangovers • Problem skin

SAFETY DATA

Non-irritant in dilution • Non-sensitizing
Slightly phototoxic – do not use in dilutions of more than 3% if going out into the sun within 12 hours of application.

Mandarin

Citrus reticulata

Family: Rutaceae

ORIGIN

Originally found in China and the Far East, the mandarin orange tree was brought over to Europe at the beginning of the nineteenth century. The fruit was a traditional offering to Chinese mandarins, and this is said to be the origin of the name. Mandarin oil is now mainly produced in the countries bordering the Mediterranean.

THERAPEUTIC PROPERTIES

Mandarin oil has similar properties to those of sweet orange. It is a 'moving' oil, useful for treating conditions where stagnation and putrefaction are present. It is a pleasant addition to a wide range of massage and bath oil blends, and may also be used to fragrance a room. Mandarin blends well with citrus oils, spice oils and clary sage, geranium, juniper, lavender and neroli.

The lack of toxicity of mandarin oil makes it very suitable for children. It has a calming and soothing effect on restless children and may be used to treat hyperactivity. It can also be beneficial in the treatment of stress, nervous tension and insomnia.

The primary action of mandarin is on the digestive system, and it can be used to treat problems arising from a slow digestion such as dyspepsia and gastralgia; it will encourage peristalsis and help to relieve constipation. As a mild digestive tonic it is useful in the treatment of the elderly. It is also suitable for treating hiccoughs, indigestion or colic in children. Blend in a base oil and massage over the abdomen.

Mandarin detoxifies the body and reduces cellulite. It is also used in the treatment of water retention and obesity. It can help to tone loose skin, for example, after losing weight.

The slightly astringent properties of mandarin make it good for combating oily skin and acne. It also has a role during pregnancy in preventing stretch marks; try combining it with neroli in a massage base oil.

METHOD OF EXTRACTION

Mandarin oil is machine-expressed from the peel of the ripe fruit.

DESCRIPTION

Mandarin oil has an extremely sweet smell with a rich, floral undertone. It is an orange or amber colour.

PSYCHOLOGICAL PROFILE

Mandarin is appropriate if you have a tendency to feel sorry for yourself. Children needing mandarin may cry a lot and tend to be restless and hard to please. You may crave comfort and seek love and attention. If you do not get the affection you crave you may overeat as compensation. Using mandarin will encourage you to be more positive about your own attributes and strengths and will help you develop a greater sense of self-worth.

OTHER VARIETIES

The mandarin tree was taken from Europe to the USA in the middle of the nineteenth century, where it was renamed tangerine by the Americans. Although the tree is still classified as *Citrus reticulata,* the tangerine has developed into a larger fruit than the mandarin and has a thinner and more citrus smell. The therapeutic properties of tangerine are similar to those of mandarin.

MOST COMMON USES

Indigestion • Restless children
Stretch marks

SAFETY DATA

Non-toxic • Non-phototoxic • Non-irritant • Non-sensitizing

Myrrh

Commiphora myrrha

Family: Burseraceae

ORIGIN

Myrrh is the resin of a small tree that grows in East Africa, countries bordering the Red Sea and Arabia. It has been used since ancient times in Egypt for the embalming of the dead and in China as a medicine for arthritis and skin infections. It has also been greatly valued as a sacred herb and incense ingredient. Distillation of the oil occurs mainly in Europe and the USA.

THERAPEUTIC PROPERTIES

Myrrh oil is stimulating, strengthening and highly antiseptic. It may be used in massage blends, steam inhalations and room fragrancing. It blends particularly well with spice oils, cedarwood, cypress, frankincense, lemon, patchouli and sandalwood.

The main action is on the respiratory system, where its tonifying properties make it helpful in the treatment of chronic lung conditions. It is also an excellent expectorant, particularly when there is thick, white mucus. It can be used to treat coughs, colds and bronchitis, where it works particularly well in steam inhalations.

The stimulating properties of myrrh also have an effect on the digestive system, where it is appropriate for treating poor digestion, fermentation and flatulence. It can also be used to cure diarrhoea from a chill; combine with other appropriate oils and massage over the abdomen.

Myrrh has a very good reputation for its action on the mouth and throat. Combined with lavender and sage in a little alcohol and water, it makes an excellent antiseptic mouthwash for any infection or inflammation in this area, including mouth ulcers, pyorrhoea, sore throat, bleeding gums, bad breath and thrush.

Myrrh has traditionally been regarded as a skin preserver, capable of delaying wrinkles and other signs of ageing skin. It combines well with frankincense, cypress, cedarwood and sandalwood for skin care. Its highly

METHOD OF EXTRACTION

The myrrh resin is gathered by making incisions in the bark. The lumps of resin are then steam-distilled to produce the essential oil.

anti-inflammatory and antiseptic properties make it a very useful oil for the treatment of any wound that is slow to heal or is infected – apply as a lotion or compress. It has also been used to treat ulcers, gangrene and fungal infections such as ringworm.

PSYCHOLOGICAL PROFILE

Myrrh is appropriate if you are a purposeful and creative person but lack confidence in your ability to overcome difficulties and achieve what you want to. You may feel temporarily in the dark, or that

DESCRIPTION

Myrrh oil is a sticky liquid ranging from a pale orange or amber colour to a dark red. It has a balsamic, medicinal and dry smell with an initial sweetness.

you are struggling with a part of your own personality.

Using myrrh will put you back in touch with your inner sense of purpose and help to open up the channels for the expression of love.

MOST COMMON USES

Mouth ulcers • Gum disease
Coughs • Ageing skin
Skin infections

Resin granules and essential oil

SAFETY DATA

Non-toxic externally • Non-irritant • Non-sensitizing

Coriander

Coriandrum sativum

Family: Umbelliferae

ORIGIN

The fruits (usually called seeds) of coriander have been used for thousands of years and were found in the tomb of the Ancient Egyptian pharaoh Rameses II. They have been used medicinally as a remedy for digestive disorders in the West and in China. It is thought that coriander is native to the Far East but became naturalized in south-eastern Europe. It was introduced into Britain by the Romans. The leaves (herb) and the fruits (spice) are popular culinary ingredients in many parts of the world. The oil is mainly produced in Russia, Eastern Europe and North Africa.

THERAPEUTIC PROPERTIES

Coriander is a gently stimulating and tonifying oil, mildly warming in effect. It makes a good addition to massage blends and may also be added to bath oils and room fragrancers. Coriander oil blends well with bergamot, clary sage, frankincense, jasmine, sandalwood and other spice oils.

Its gently tonifying action on the nervous system makes coriander helpful in cases of debility. It is said to improve a poor memory, and can alleviate migraine, especially if this is associated with digestive symptoms; add to a massage blend or the bath.

The main action of coriander is on the digestive system, which is why it features as an ingredient in many aperitifs and liqueurs. It is an excellent digestive tonic, encouraging better assimilation, and is an important oil in the treatment of anorexia nervosa, helping to stimulate the appetite, improve an undermined digestion and strengthen the nervous system. Other digestive disorders that coriander oil can treat include colic, diarrhoea, dyspepsia, flatulence and nausea. To relieve digestive discomfort, blend coriander into a base oil with other appropriate essential oils and massage over the abdomen.

METHOD OF EXTRACTION

The fruits are crushed and the oil is then steam-distilled.

DESCRIPTION

Coriander oil has a fresh, aromatic and sweet-spicy smell. It is a colourless or pale yellow liquid.

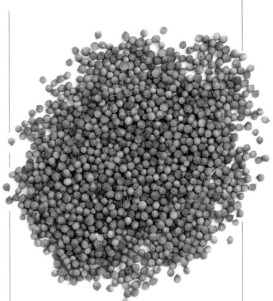

Coriander is also known to have aphrodisiac properties. It is particularly appropriate when the libido is low as a result of tiredness and debility. Add to a massage or bath oil blend with other aphrodisiac oils or use to fragrance the room.

Coriander has an analgesic and warming effect, making it a helpful addition to blends treating rheumatic pains, muscular stiffness, sprains and strains and neuralgia. It is also an effective deodorant in that it both masks unpleasant smells and prevents the growth of bacteria that cause body odour. Blend it into lotions and flower waters to use as deodorants, colognes and body splashes.

Psychological profile

Coriander is appropriate if you present a misleading appearance; you may seem confident, independent and even arrogant, but underneath you are a rather needy and clingy person who does not actually like yourself. You probably feel that your parents had high expectations of you and that you now have similarly high expectations of yourself, but are having difficulty living up to them. This split between how you feel and what you show to the world may lead to depression, eating disorders and feelings of desperation. Using coriander oil will bring a feeling of comfort and inner strength that will help you to come to terms with who you really are and begin to express the vulnerable side of your nature.

MOST COMMON USES

Anorexia • Poor digestion
Rheumatism • Deodorant

Safety data

Non-toxic • Non-irritant in dilution • Non-sensitizing

Cypress

Cupressus sempervirens

Family: Cupressaceae

ORIGIN

Cypress trees are native to the countries bordering the Mediterranean. Cypress has been used as an astringent herbal medicine since ancient times and is valued greatly in Tibet as an incense ingredient. Cultivation and distillation occur mainly in France and Morocco. The oil is used as a fragrance ingredient in many aftershaves and colognes.

THERAPEUTIC PROPERTIES

Cypress's main characteristic is its astringent properties and its main action is on the circulatory system. Cypress may be used in massage and bath oil blends, in steam inhalations and room fragrancing. It blends particularly well with cedarwood, clary sage, frankincense, juniper, lavender, mandarin, marjoram and orange.

Cypress refreshes and tones the nervous system. It may be used to treat nervous debility, nervous strain and weariness brought about by stress.

Cypress is very useful in the treatment of varicose veins or broken capillaries; dilute in a base oil and massage over the affected area. It is the main oil for treating haemorrhoids; try adding a couple of drops to the bath. Cypress combines well with ginger and may be massaged on to the hands or feet or used in a footbath to treat poor circulation and chilblains.

The astringent properties of cypress make it good for treating excessive discharges; it can be used for hot and burning diarrhoea, frequent urination and most forms of haemorrhage. To stop a nosebleed, put a couple of drops of cypress on a tissue and hold under the nose for a few moments.

Cypress has a tonifying effect on uterine and pelvic tissue and can relieve heavy and prolonged menstrual bleeding. It can be helpful during the menopause and

METHOD OF EXTRACTION

The oil is extracted by steam distillation of the needles and twigs.

DESCRIPTION

Cypress oil is pale yellow or green in colour and has a sweet, resinous, fresh odour reminiscent of a pine forest.

PSYCHOLOGICAL PROFILE

Cypress works best for those people who tend towards excess and over-indulgence. Such people may be lazy and overweight and perhaps of an easy-going and chatty nature. If appropriate, cypress will help to focus and increase your energy.

will relieve hot flushes; use in the bath and as a massage oil.

Cypress can help to relieve muscular aches and pains. It may be used as a compress or massage oil to relieve rheumatism. It will reduce swelling and oedema of the joints.

This oil has a detoxifying effect on the system. It helps to prevent the build-up of excess fluid and toxins within the tissues and may be used in the treatment of water retention, obesity and cellulite. Use in massage and bath oils.

Cypress is suitable for oily skin and also for areas of loose skin, for example, after losing weight. It may be used as a facial steam or in a massage oil or lotion. It will also help to check excessive perspiration and is a natural deodorant; foot baths with cypress and lavender oil are an effective way to deal with foot odour.

Cypress also has antispasmodic properties and can be used in steam inhalations to relieve spasmodic and loose coughs, hayfever, bronchitis and asthma.

MOST COMMON USES

Varicose veins and haemorrhoids
Poor circulation • Heavy periods
Profuse perspiration
Spasmodic coughs

SAFETY DATA

Non-toxic • Non-irritant • Non-sensitizing

Lemongrass

Cymbopogon citratus, C. flexuosus

Family: Gramineae

ORIGIN

*There are two main types of lemongrass: West Indian lemongrass (**Cymbopogon citratus**) and East Indian lemongrass (**Cymbopogon flexuosus**). Both varieties are native to India, although the former is now mainly cultivated in the Caribbean. Lemongrass is a fast-growing, aromatic perennial grass that grows up to 1.5 m (5 ft) tall. It is used in India to treat fevers and infectious illnesses and appears as a culinary herb throughout Asia.*

THERAPEUTIC PROPERTIES

Lemongrass has the refreshing and antiseptic properties of lemon but is more warming. It should be well diluted (do not use in concentrations of more than 2%) and may be used in massage oils, insect-repellent preparations and room fragrancing. Lemongrass blends particularly well with coriander, eucalyptus, lavender, peppermint, rosemary, thyme and vetiver.

The main actions of lemongrass are on the digestive system and skin. It is also a mild antidepressant and will relieve stress and nervous exhaustion.

Lemongrass will help to stimulate the appetite and tone a sluggish digestive system. It has been used to treat colitis and because of its antiseptic properties it is helpful for enteritis and other gastric infections. Combine with geranium in a base oil and massage over the abdomen.

The tonifying properties of lemongrass are beneficial for poor muscle tone and slack tissues. It is an excellent component for any sports oil blend, both for a pre-sport massage and to treat aching muscles or muscle strain after sports. Combine with rosemary and vetiver in a base oil and massage into muscles before and after sport.

Lemongrass has a tonifying, deodorizing and astringent effect on the skin. It can be used to treat open or blocked

METHOD OF EXTRACTION

Lemongrass essential oil is produced by steam distillation of the chopped grass. After distillation the exhausted grass is used as cattle feed.

DESCRIPTION

Lemongrass essential oil has a fresh, intensely sweet, lemony and herbaceous smell and is a pale yellow or amber liquid.

pores and acne, and may be added to a facial steam to deep-cleanse the skin.

This oil is widely used as an insect repellent for mosquitoes and fleas. It is also a parasiticide, eliminating lice, scabies and ticks.

PSYCHOLOGICAL PROFILE

Lemongrass is appropriate if you feel you have been a victim of circumstances or other people's behaviour during your life. You may be someone who is easily used and taken for granted by other people and you find it difficult to assert yourself or to free yourself from restrictions. Using lemongrass will help you to become aware that there may be other ways of responding to your situation, and then new possibilities will begin to open up for you.

OTHER VARIETIES

Another variety of *Cymbopogon* used in aromatherapy is *C. nardus*, or citronella. Citronella oil is mainly used as an insect repellent, particularly against mosquitoes. Dilute in a base oil or flower water and apply to exposed areas of skin, or use in an essential oil burner in a room.

MOST COMMON USES

Enteritis • Acne • Sports preparation
Insect repellent • Parasiticide

SAFETY DATA

Non-toxic • Avoid use on hypersensitive or damaged skin
Do not use in more than 2% concentration

Palmarosa

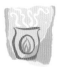

Cymbopogon martinii var. martinii

Family: Gramineae

ORIGIN

Palmarosa is a grassy-leaved herbaceous plant of the same family as lemongrass and citronella. It is native to India but is now also cultivated, and the oil produced, in Indonesia, the Comoros Islands, East Africa and Brazil. The essential oil is used in perfumery, particularly in soap, and was frequently employed in the past to adulterate the more expensive rose oil.

THERAPEUTIC PROPERTIES

Palmarosa is a cooling and tonifying oil with healing and regenerative properties similar to those of lavender, and is also a balancing oil, being both calming and uplifting. A pleasant oil to use, palmarosa may be added to massage blends, bath oils and room fragrancers. Palmarosa oil combines well with rose, bergamot, cedarwood, geranium, mandarin, sandalwood and ylang ylang.

This oil has a soothing and mildly strengthening effect on the nervous system and is useful in the treatment of stress, anxiety and nervous tension. It has a mild aphrodisiac effect and is helpful where stress and tension are getting in the way of sexual fulfilment.

The action of palmarosa on the digestive system is as a gentle tonic and aid to digestion and assimilation. It will help to improve the appetite and may be used in the treatment of anorexia nervosa. Palmarosa is an effective antiseptic in the treatment of diarrhoea, gastroenteritis and dysentery; try combining it with bergamot and geranium. It will help to rebalance the intestinal flora after an intestinal infection or a course of antibiotics: use as a massage oil and massage over the abdomen or add to a bath oil blend.

Palmarosa is best known for its skin care properties. It has a balancing action on the skin and can help to hydrate dry skin and balance the sebum secretions of oily skin. It will

METHOD OF EXTRACTION

The essential oil is steam- or water-distilled from the fresh or dried grass. Palmarosa oil is frequently adulterated by the similar but inferior oil of gingergrass (*Cymbopogon martinii var. sofia*).

DESCRIPTION

*Palmarosa oil is a pale yellow
or pale green liquid with a sweet,
rosy, floral smell.*

reduce scar tissue and its antiseptic
properties are helpful for acne and
minor skin infections. Palmarosa
stimulates cellular regeneration and
will reduce wrinkles and improve the
appearance of tired or ageing skin; it
may also be used to help prevent
stretch marks. Apply to the skin in
massage oils, compresses, creams and
lotions and use as a facial steam.

PSYCHOLOGICAL PROFILE

Palmarosa is most appropriate if you
tend to live in the past and do not feel
optimistic about the future. You may
feel that your life has not worked out
how you wanted it to and you are
disappointed and depressed. You may
also fear the ageing process. It may be
that you have experienced a particular
crisis, such as losing your job or your
partner, or there may be a more
gradual feeling that life never fulfilled
the expectations of your younger days.
Using palmarosa will help you to feel
more optimistic about your present life
and to get more in touch with your
inner sense of worth.

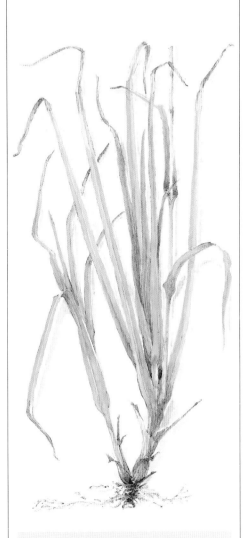

MOST COMMON USES

Stress • Diarrhoea • Skin care

SAFETY DATA

Non-toxic • Non-irritant • Non-sensitizing

Cardamom

Elettaria cardamomum

Family: Zingiberaceae

ORIGIN

The seeds and pods of cardamom have been used for centuries as a culinary spice in India, its native country. Cardamom has been employed in traditional Chinese medicine and in Indian Ayurvedic medicine for over 3000 years, primarily for the treatment of respiratory diseases, fevers and digestive complaints. The essential oil also has a long history of use and has been produced since the sixteenth century. Cardamom oil is a perfume ingredient, especially in oriental-type fragrances. The oil is now produced mainly in India, Europe and the USA.

THERAPEUTIC PROPERTIES

Cardamom is a warming and restorative oil which has a tonifying and calming action on the nervous system. It is pleasant to use in massage blends and combines particularly well with bergamot, cedarwood, clove, frankincense, orange, sandalwood and ylang ylang.

The restorative properties of cardamom make it useful in the treatment of mental fatigue – try combining it with rosemary and burning it in the room. It will also relieve nervous tension. Cardamom has aphrodisiac properties, useful where feelings of stress and tension are getting in the way of sexual enjoyment. It is particularly helpful in the treatment of impotence. Combine with other appropriate oils such as jasmine or sandalwood and use in massage or burn in the room.

The main action of cardamom is on the digestive system: it is antispasmodic and carminative and will alleviate nausea, flatulence, indigestion, colic and heartburn. It may be diluted in a base oil and massaged over the abdomen, or the seed may be chewed to release the essential oil. It can be used as a general tonic for a sluggish digestive system and help to encourage better assimilation of food. It is also used in the treatment of anorexia. Cardamom is an important oil in the

METHOD OF EXTRACTION

Cardamom essential oil is steam-distilled from the dried seeds.

treatment of headaches related to digestive disorders. Use in massage blends and in the bath.

The antiseptic properties of cardamom make it a good addition to mouthwashes for the treatment of bad breath. Try combining it with myrrh and lavender and diluting in alcohol and water for use as a mouthwash.

DESCRIPTION

The oil is colourless to pale yellow and has a sweet-spicy, aromatic smell with a woody and almost floral undertone.

PSYCHOLOGICAL PROFILE

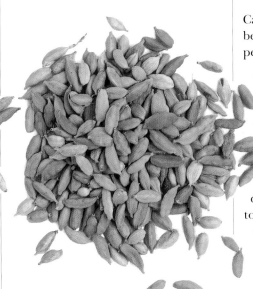

Cardamom is appropriate if you have become a dry and melancholic type of person. You probably have a sedentary job and tend to have an intellectual approach to life, disliking excessive displays of emotion. You tend to be a rather fearful person and are anxious about your health. Other people may find you over-critical and rather unapproachable. Using cardamom will help you to get back in touch with the feeling of joy and encourage you to express greater warmth and friendliness with others.

MOST COMMON USES

Digestive tonic • Nausea • Heartburn
Poor assimilation • Bad breath

SAFETY DATA

Non-toxic • Non-irritant • Non-sensitizing

Eucalyptus

Eucalyptus globulus
Family: Myrtaceae

ORIGIN

The eucalyptus or blue gum tree is indigenous to Australia and was used as a medicinal herb by the Aborigines. In the nineteenth century a German botanist, von Muller, introduced the tree and its essential oil to the rest of the world. It is now cultivated in North Africa, Spain, California and India as well as Australia.

THERAPEUTIC PROPERTIES

Eucalyptus is a warming and drying oil with excellent antiseptic properties. It may be used in massage blends and bath oils and is especially effective as a steam inhalation. It blends particularly well with cedarwood, cypress, lavender, lemon, marjoram, pine, tea tree and thyme.

Eucalyptus has a refreshing effect on the nervous system and may be used to treat tiredness, poor concentration, headaches and debility. Use in inhalations or burn in the room.

The Australian Aborigines used eucalyptus in the treatment of all kinds of fever, including malaria. The essential oil is especially good for infections of the respiratory tract such as colds, flu, sinusitis, bronchitis and pneumonia. Because it is a warming oil it works especially well if you are feeling chilled. It is also decongestant and makes an excellent inhalation to relieve over-production of mucus, especially thick white mucus. It can be combined with aniseed to treata a cough or cypress to treat catarrh. Eucalyptus may also be used to treat asthma.

Eucalyptus is an important remedy for the treatment of rheumatism and arthritis, especially when there is a lot of stiffness and loss of mobility and the symptoms are worse when it is cold and damp. Try combining it with lavender and pine and using as a compress or massage lotion.

As an antibiotic oil eucalyptus can be used to treat infections of the urinary tract, especially if there is pus in the urine. Try it when cystitis is brought on by a chill. It is also good for genital

METHOD OF EXTRACTION

Eucalyptus oil is extracted by steam distillation of the leaves and young twigs.

DESCRIPTION

A clear or pale yellow liquid, eucalyptus has a strong medicinal-camphoraceous smell and a faint woody undertone.

infections such as leucorrhoea; dilute it well and use in a sitz bath.

The antibiotic properties of eucalyptus make it helpful in the treatment of skin infections and wounds, herpes and ulcers. It may be dabbed directly on to the skin to relieve the pain or itching of insect bites and stings. Eucalyptus is also a parasiticide and may be combined with other oils to remove lice. It is anti-fungal and may

MOST COMMON USES

Colds and flu • Bronchitis
Mucus congestion/sinusitis
Rheumatism • Cystitis
Infectious diseases • Insect repellent

be used to treat athlete's foot and other fungal infections.

Eucalyptus oil makes an excellent antiseptic room spray to fumigate a sickroom. It is also an effective insect repellent, especially if combined with cypress and lemon.

PSYCHOLOGICAL PROFILE

Eucalyptus is indicated if you recognize that it is time for a change in your life, but feel bogged down. You will feel restless, but have become trapped by fear of change and a lack of direction. This in turn leads to a state of confusion. Eucalyptus will allow you to gain clarity and move forward in your life, cutting through the fear and confusion.

OTHER VARIETIES

Eucalyptus citriodora is also highly antiseptic but is more cooling in its action than *E. globulus*. It has a pleasant lemony smell. Use this variety for respiratory infections where the mucus secretions are yellow, indicating there is heat in the system. *E. citriodora* is also useful for rheumatism when the joints are hot and red.

SAFETY DATA

Non-toxic externally • Toxic internally • Non-irritant • Non-sensitizing

Fennel

Foeniculum vulgare var. dulce

Also known as: Sweet fennel

Family: Umbelliferae

ORIGIN

There are many cultivated varieties of fennel, all of them related to wild fennel, which is native to the countries bordering the Mediterranean. The variety used in aromatherapy is sweet fennel, which is cultivated in France, Italy and Greece. Fennel has been used as a sacred and medicinal herb for thousands of years. It was believed to ward off evil spirits and impart longevity, courage and strength.

THERAPEUTIC PROPERTIES

Fennel oil is primarily a 'moving' or unblocking oil and its main action is on the digestive system. It may be used in massage blends and inhalations, but not at concentrations of more than 1.5% as there may be some toxicity in concentrated doses. It blends particularly well with geranium, lavender, marjoram and rose.

A calminative and digestive stimulant, fennel will relieve flatulence and digestive spasms. When food is not properly carried through the digestive system, putrefaction occurs and gas will form; fennel is one of the main oils to encourage food to be digested properly and to help expel gas. It may be combined with a tiny amount of cinnamon and massaged over the abdomen to stimulate and strengthen the digestion.

Fennel is similar in action and smell to aniseed, but aniseed works more on the upper digestive tract and stomach while the action of fennel is more on the lower digestive processes and bowel. Fennel can be used to relieve constipation; dilute in a carrier oil and massage over the abdomen. It is also useful in the treatment of nervous indigestion such as is brought on by hurrying or after an emotional upset. It is the main oil for treating a swollen

METHOD OF EXTRACTION

The essential oil is steam-distilled from crushed fennel seeds.

distended abdomen and will relieve bloating after a rich or large meal.

Fennel oil also has an important action on the lungs. It is a mild expectorant and will help to relieve a phlegmy cough. Combine with other appropriate oils in a base oil and use in a chest rub, or burn in the room.

Fennel is a diuretic and increases the loss of fluids from the body. It can be used in a massage blend to detoxify the body, for example when treating cellulite. It has an oestrogenic action on the body and can help to increase milk production in nursing mothers. It may also help to relieve engorged or painful breasts; use as a compress.

Fennel oil has been shown to be effective at eliminating lactobacillus, which is thought to be the main bacterium that causes tooth decay. This indicates the usefulness of fennel in dental preparations, such as toothpastes and mouthwashes. Fennel will also help to mask unpleasant odours.

PSYCHOLOGICAL PROFILE

Fennel will be of most benefit to you if you are the type of person who holds back from expressing yourself. This may be as a result of a repressive childhood, and inadequate opportunity to communicate deep emotions. This can result in a lack of enthusiasm, a fear of communicating

DESCRIPTION

Fennel oil is a pale yellow colour and has a sweet-spicy, green smell reminiscent of aniseed.

and little opportunity to experience and learn. The habit of withholding expression on the emotional level can lead to flatulence and constipation physically. If appropriate, fennel can help you to relax and be more open to the experience of life.

OTHER VARIETIES

Bitter fennel (*Foeniculum vulgare var. amara*) is also available as an essential oil. It shares many of the medicinal virtues of sweet fennel but is harsher and more likely to cause sensitization. It is advisable to use only sweet fennel for aromatherapy.

MOST COMMON USES

Flatulence • Constipation
Nervous indigestion • Bloatedness
Phlegmy coughs

SAFETY DATA

Sensitization possible • Do not use in concentrations of more than 1.5%

Star anise

Illicium verum

Also known as: Star aniseed, Chinese anise

Family: Illiciaceae

ORIGIN

Star anise is the fruit of an evergreen tree native to China. It has been used as a culinary spice and medicine for the treatment of digestive disorders and coughs for millenia. In the East, aniseed (which has similar properties) is often chewed after meals to sweeten the breath and aid digestion. Today, production of the essential oil takes place mainly in China and India.

THERAPEUTIC PROPERTIES

Star anise is a calming and sedating oil that is useful for relieving mental and physical tension. It should not be used in concentrations of more than 2%, and not at all on people with hypersensitive or damaged skin, or on infants under two years of age.

When diluted, star anise may be used for massage or as an inhalation. It combines particularly well with chamomile, cinnamon, clove, eucalyptus, lavender, orange, pine and rosemary essential oils.

Anise relaxes physical contraction and therefore can be used wherever there is any form of tension or spasm in the body. It will relieve hiccups, indigestion with cramping pains, nervous digestion and upwardly moving gas. It is more efficacious on the stomach than the lower digestive processes, although it can also be used for colic, flatulence and headaches of a digestive origin. To treat digestive disorders, anise should be well diluted in a base oil and massaged over the stomach or abdomen. It works particularly well when combined with chamomile. The antispasmodic properties of star anise are also helpful in relieving painful periods.

Star anise has an expectorant effect which will help to clear mucus from the lungs, for example in the case of bronchitis; try combining the oil with eucalyptus as an effective steam inhalation. Star anise also helps to

---

METHOD OF EXTRACTION

The essential oil is produced by steam distillation of the fruits.

80

DESCRIPTION

Star anise oil has an intensely sweet, clean smell reminiscent of liquorice. It ranges in colour from completely clear to very pale yellow.

strengthen the lungs, and its antispasmodic properties make it useful in treating a wide range of coughs. Use it as an inhalation at the beginning of a cold if you find that colds often settle on your chest.

The antispasmodic properties of star anise make it useful for treating muscular cramps or spasms; dilute it to use as a compress or rubbing oil. Star anise may also be blended with other appropriate oils to treat aching muscles and rheumatism.

PSYCHOLOGICAL PROFILE

Star anise has comforting and soothing properties appropriate for people who crave being comforted and soothed by others. If you are super-sensitive to the harshness of life and feel that pain and hardship are unbearable, star anise will help to calm and strengthen you.

Fruits or seeds in the star-shaped seed follicles

OTHER VARIETIES

A similar essential oil is produced from the seeds of the herb aniseed (*Pimpinella anisum*). This oil has many of the same properties as star anise but it has been known to cause dermatitis in susceptible people and so is not now widely used.

MOST COMMON USES

Antispasmodic
Colic and flatulence • Coughs

SAFETY DATA

Non-irritant in dilution • Non-sensitizing
Do not use in concentrations of more than 2%

Jasmine

Jasminum officinale

Family: Oleaceae

ORIGIN

A native of north-west India, jasmine has been highly valued for the scent of its flowers for thousands of years and is known as the 'king of perfumes' because of its importance to the fragrance industry; indeed, a whole industry grew up around it in the Grasse region of France. Because the flowers are too delicate to be steam-distilled, jasmine used to be extracted by a labour-intensive method known as enfleurage, but today the usual method is by solvent extraction (see below). Jasmine absolute is produced mainly in France, Morocco and India.

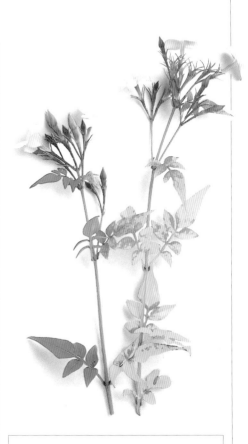

THERAPEUTIC PROPERTIES

Jasmine is the most uplifting of all the oils. Its main effect is on the emotions, where it promotes a state of relaxed awareness; wearing jasmine helps to increase self-confidence and is anti-depressant. It is at once refreshing,

METHOD OF EXTRACTION

Jasmine for aromatherapy use is not strictly speaking an essential oil but an absolute. First, a concrète is produced from jasmine flowers by a process of solvent extraction. Then the solvent is removed and the absolute is obtained from the concrète by separation with alcohol. Jasmine absolute is a very costly substance because of the large volume of flowers required to produce a small amount of it.

DESCRIPTION

Jasmine has an intensely rich, warm, heady, floral scent. It is a viscous, dark orange-brown liquid.

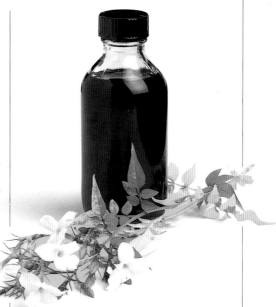

soothing and calming, most effective where there is a clear and direct link between psychological stress and physical discomfort. Its relaxing properties make jasmine a useful oil where there are symptoms of contraction, tension and blockage, for example, a tight chest or tense muscles. Jasmine blends well with bergamot, clary sage, orange, rose, sandalwood and ylang ylang.

The relaxing yet uplifting properties of jasmine suggest its use as one of the classic aphrodisiac oils, its exotic smell creating an atmosphere of relaxation and enjoyment. It can be beneficial in the treatment of both impotence and frigidity. Use as a sensual massage oil.

Jasmine will ease menstrual discomfort and cramps, and help relieve the pain of labour; it may be used either to perfume the room or diluted in a base oil to be massaged into the lower back between contractions.

In skin care, jasmine is beneficial for treating hot, dry and inflamed skin, especially if this is worse during times of emotional stress. It may be applied undiluted to the skin as a perfume.

PSYCHOLOGICAL PROFILE

Jasmine is most suitable when you are going through a time of trauma and grief. It is also appropriate if you have become trapped by lingering feelings of sadness or grief. The use of jasmine can help to encourage an acceptance of all the experiences of life and promote enjoyment and relaxation.

MOST COMMON USES

Uplifting • Aphrodisiac
Labour • Dry skin

SAFETY DATA

Non-toxic • Non-irritating • Non-sensitizing

Juniper

Juniperus communis

Family: Cupressaceae

ORIGIN

Juniper is an evergreen shrub or tree which produces small black berries. It is widespread throughout the northern hemisphere. Juniper has a long history of use as a herbal medicine in the treatment of urinary disorders, gout and rheumatism and respiratory problems. The berries are used to flavour gin.

THERAPEUTIC PROPERTIES

Juniper is a warming, stimulating and tonifying oil. It makes an excellent refreshing and detoxifying addition to many bath oils and massage oils, and may also be used in inhalations and room freshening. It blends particularly well with cedarwood, cypress, ginger, lavender, pine, rosemary and all the citrus oils.

The main action of juniper is on the kidneys and urinary system. It can be appropriate for both excessive and diminished urination and is one of the most important oils in the treatment of cystitis, especially when this is worse in cold weather.

Juniper will encourage the elimination of uric acid and other toxins that a cold, sluggish system may fail to excrete efficiently. For this reason it is known as a blood purifier. It combines well with cypress to treat fluid retention, obesity and cellulite, and can also be used in the treatment of urinary stones (use in compresses over the lower back) and gout (use in footbaths or compresses). Juniper is an important oil in the treatment of rheumatism and arthritis, especially in cases that are worse in cold weather. Combine it with a rubbing oil and massage over the affected parts or use in a compress.

This is a good oil for tonifying the glandular system, particularly the adrenals and pancreas – use it in

METHOD OF EXTRACTION

Juniper oil is steam-distilled from the berries alone or from the berries, needles and twigs of the shrub. Distillation occurs mainly in France and eastern Europe.

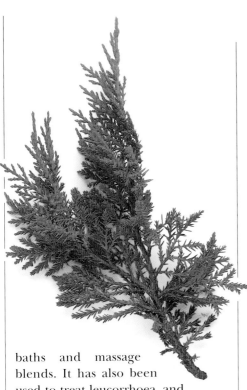

Juniper oil has a piercing, fresh, warm, woody-herbaceous smell. The oil from the berries is slightly sweeter and less harsh than that from the wood, needles and twigs. It is a colourless or pale yellow liquid.

The stimulating, astringent and detoxifying properties of juniper make it a good oil to treat clogged, oily and unhealthy skin. It will help the body to remove impurities and will improve skin that is prone to blackheads and acne. A few drops of juniper oil make an excellent, deep-cleansing steam facial. It can also be used to treat weeping eczema and dermatitis.

PSYCHOLOGICAL PROFILE

Juniper is appropriate if you were misunderstood and lonely in childhood. You may have appeared shy and, from fear of rejection, kept to yourself. In later life this may have developed into aloofness and a lack of the ability to give and receive warmth and affection. The lack of emotional care as a child may also develop into a neglect in looking after yourself physically. The use of juniper will promote a more optimistic outlook and encourage a warmer and friendlier state of being.

baths and massage blends. It has also been used to treat leucorrhoea, and absent, painful or scanty periods. It used to be thought that juniper oil should be avoided by pregnant women, because juniper berries taken internally can cause miscarriage, but in fact juniper oil used externally is not abortifacient and is safe to use at normal dilutions during pregnancy.

MOST COMMON USES

Cystitis • Water retention • Cellulite
Rheumatism • Oily skin • Acne

SAFETY DATA

Non-toxic • Non-irritant in dilution • Non-sensitizing

Lavender

***Lavandula angustifolia,
syn. L. officinalis, L. vera***

Family: Labiatae

ORIGIN

An aromatic shrub native to the Mediterranean region, lavender has a long history of use as a medicine, fragrance and insect repellent. The essential oil production is long-established in the Provence region of France and also occurs in many other countries.

THERAPEUTIC PROPERTIES

This is the most versatile and well-used of all the essential oils, its lack of toxicity making it a valuable remedy for everyday use. It may be used in massage blends, bath oils, room fragrancing, compresses, douches and steam inhalations, and is one of the few essential oils that may be applied to the skin without dilution.

Lavender is a balancing or regulating oil. In the long run it does tend towards sedating or calming, although initially it has a reviving effect – a footbath with a few drops of lavender added has one of the most restorative effects imaginable. Like jasmine, it can be used to treat any physical symptoms that are the result of stress or nervous tension.

Lavender is relaxing as it calms cerebro-spinal activity. It may be used to treat irritability, depression, insomnia, hysteria, shock and nervous tension. It also has mild analgesic properties, which make it an important oil in the treatment of headaches and migraine, and good for all forms of neuralgia, shingles, sciatica, muscular pains and rheumatism. It will relieve earache in children; massage a few drops around the ear.

Its restorative and calming effect on the heart means that it is helpful for high blood pressure and palpitations – use it in massage and bath preparations, and as an inhalant to relieve fainting and shock.

The antispasmodic properties of lavender make it efficacious in the treatment of any kind of spasmodic cough. The excellent antiseptic properties are effective in treating flu, bronchitis and pneumonia.

METHOD OF EXTRACTION

Lavender oil is steam-distilled from the fresh flowering tops of the plant.

Lavender may be used to treat colic and flatulence. It is of most benefit when treating digestive problems with a nervous origin, including diarrhoea, indigestion, nausea and so on. Dilute in a base oil and massage into the abdomen.

The anti-bacterial and anti-inflammatory properties of lavender have a pronounced effect on the urinary system and genitals – use in the bath. It is excellent for treating cystitis, leucorrhoea, thrush and other genital infections. The anti-spasmodic properties can soothe menstrual cramps.

Lavender is extremely useful in a variety of skin conditions, including wounds, ulcers and sores of all kinds. As a first-aid remedy it can be used neat on abrasions, wounds, burns, insect bites and stings. Other skin conditions that lavender may help are dermatitis, eczema, acne, acne rosaceae, psoriasis and scarring.

MOST COMMON USES

Stress and tension • Insomnia
Headaches • Neuralgia
First-aid – wounds, burns, shock
Insect repellent • Thrush

DESCRIPTION

A colourless or pale yellow liquid, lavender oil has a very familiar, fresh, floral, slightly harsh and sweet smell.

Combined with lemon and used as a compress, it will treat boils. Lavender may be combined with other oils to eliminate lice and scabies and to repel mosquitoes. Its deodorizing properties make it a useful room spray and antiseptic and a good addition to a mouthwash.

PSYCHOLOGICAL PROFILE

If you are a sensitive person who is easily embarrassed and inhibited you need lavender. You may have learnt to conceal your shyness by appearing to be efficient, practical and organized, yet behind this you are aware of your sensitivity and vulnerability to other people. Using lavender will help you to accept your sensitivity and make the most of new situations that so often leave you feeling frustrated and unable to express yourself.

SAFETY DATA

Non-toxic • Non-irritant • Non-sensitizing

Chamomile

Matricaria recutica*, syn. *M. chamomilla

Also known as: Blue chamomile, German chamomile

Family: Compositae

ORIGIN

Chamomile is a flowering herb that has been used medicinally for thousands of years. The flowers are taken as an infusion for digestive disorders and to treat nervous tension and insomnia. Chamomile is cultivated in central and northern Europe.

THERAPEUTIC PROPERTIES

Chamomile is a profoundly soothing and calming oil. The main effects of chamomile are on the nervous and digestive systems. It is widely used in massage blends, skin care creams and bath oils, and blends particularly well with clary sage, lavender, lemon, marjoram and rose.

Chamomile is suitable for treating any digestive complaint arising from a nervous origin, including colic, indigestion and peptic ulcers. Because of its low toxicity it is suitable for treating children's digestive upsets, such as diarrhoea or colic. It combines well with star anise when treating digestive problems.

The pain-relieving properties of chamomile make it excellent for treating teething pains in infants, especially when combined with fretfulness or earache. Chamomile also stimulates leucocyte (white blood cell) production and is useful when treating any kind of virus or infection, especially in children.

Its antispasmodic properties make it a good treatment for menstrual cramp, and it is a mild emmenagogue, bringing on a menstrual period delayed due to cold or emotional upset. It is very soothing for genital irritation, particularly vaginal pruritis. Chamomile compresses can be excellent in relieving the pain and inflammation of mastitis, especially when combined with lavender or rose. It can be helpful during the menopause for menstrual irregularities, especially when associated with irritability or nervous complaints. Try blending it with rose and using for massage and in the bath.

METHOD OF EXTRACTION

Chamomile oil is produced by steam distillation of the flowers.

Chamomile has a very calming and sedative effect on the nervous system, helping to relieve insomnia, irritability and nervousness. Combined with lavender or geranium and massaged over the site, it will help to relieve the pain of neuralgia or sciatica. It soothes inflamed joints and aching muscles and may also help to relieve tension headaches.

One of the most important uses of chamomile is in treating skin inflammation; its anti-inflammatory and soothing properties make it particularly appropriate for allergic skin conditions. It may also be used to treat eczema, rashes, herpes, wounds, irritation, dryness and any stress-related skin condition. For skin care, use chamomile in the bath, in a lotion or as a compress.

DESCRIPTION

A deep ink-blue viscous liquid that becomes brown with age, chamomile oil has an intensely heavy, sweet and herbaceous smell with a fruity undertone.

MOST COMMON USES

Colic • Menstrual cramps • Neuralgia
Inflammation • Eczema and allergies

PSYCHOLOGICAL PROFILE

Children needing chamomile are nervous and sensitive; adults requiring it feel misunderstood, and most likely are, because they tend to hide their inner sensitivity under a layer of defensive behaviour, irritability and emotional over-reaction. Using chamomile oil will help to soothe your reactions and calm your nervousness, enabling you to express your sensitivity.

OTHER VARIETIES

Roman chamomile, distilled from the flowers of *Anthemis nobilis*, is pale yellow and has a milder, sweeter smell than blue chamomile. Roman chamomile shares all the therapeutic properties of blue chamomile but is milder in effect and is particularly suitable for treating infants or people with a weak constitution.

SAFETY DATA

Non-toxic • Non-irritant • Non-sensitizing

Tea tree

Melaleuca alternifolia

Also known as: Ti tree

Family: Myrtaceae

ORIGIN

*This species of the **Melaleuca** family is native to Australia. Tea tree has been used for thousands of years by the Australian Aborigines, who crush the leaves and use them to treat infected wounds and skin problems. During the Second World War, it was included in first-aid kits to treat infections.*

THERAPEUTIC PROPERTIES

Tea tree is a stimulating and tonifying oil used primarily for its germicidal properties. It is highly antiseptic and can combat many different kinds of bacterial infection, including streptococcal and staphylococcal types, and has also been shown to have significant anti-viral and anti-fungal properties. In addition, it has the ability to stimulate the immune response and actually works more effectively when there are signs of infection present. It blends particularly well with other strongly antiseptic oils, such as clove, eucalyptus, lavender, lemon, pine, rosemary and thyme.

Tea tree oil is used to treat many kinds of respiratory tract infections. It is extremely useful in helping to throw off colds and flu, and works particularly well in a steam inhalation.

Another important area of action for tea tree oil is the genito-urinary tract. It is effective for both acute and chronic cystitis and has become one of the main treatments for many genital infections, including thrush, non-specific urethritis (NSU), genital herpes, genital warts, pruritis and trichomonas. Due to its low toxicity, it can safely be used in high concentration in baths and can be applied in pessaries.

As an excellent anti-fungal, tea tree can be applied locally to treat such conditions as athlete's foot and ringworm. It is widely used in lotions to treat acne and is also a mild analgesic, bringing relief of pain as well as combating infection in ailments such as corns, callouses, whitlows, boils, wounds, cuts and burns. To disinfect

METHOD OF EXTRACTION

Tea tree oil is steam- or water-distilled from the leaves and twigs of the tree.

A colourless or pale yellow liquid, tea tree oil has a strong, spicy, fresh-camphoraceous smell.

a cut or soothe insect stings and bites, apply tea tree neat – it will not even sting.

Tea tree can be mixed with water and alcohol and used as a mouthwash to treat bad breath, mouth ulcers and gum infections. Many cases of warts and verrucae have been eliminated by the use of tea tree oil – try dabbing it on neat on a daily basis. Tea tree is also effective in the treatment of cold sores and other types of herpes.

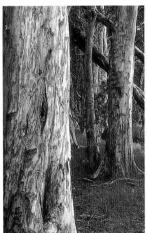

Cajuput trees (M. leucodendron)

PSYCHOLOGICAL PROFILE

Although tea tree will work effectively for a wide range of first-aid and acute ailments, it is most appropriate if you are prone to complaints that are lingering and slow to heal. You may also have the feeling that you are never quite reaching your full potential, and that you are somehow disadvantaged and held back by circumstances beyond your control. Using tea tree will help you to realize that you can have an effect on your life and that you can take at least the next step towards a more fulfilling, happy and purposeful existence.

OTHER VARIETIES

There are two other types of *Melaleuca* that share the strongly antiseptic and stimulating properties of tea tree. Niaouli (*M. viridiflora*), also native to Australia, is primarily used in the treatment of respiratory illnesses such as bronchitis, asthma and catarrh. It can also be used in steam inhalations for treating acute infections such as colds, flu, rhinitis and sinusitis. Cajuput (*M. leucodendron*) is native to Indonesia and the Philippines and is used in the same way as niaouli in the treatment of respiratory conditions.

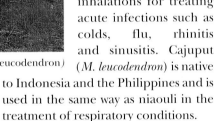

MOST COMMON USES

Anti-bacterial • Anti-viral • Anti-fungal
Colds and flu • Cystitis • Thrush • Herpes
First-aid • Skin infections

SAFETY DATA

Non-toxic externally • Non-irritant • Skin sensitization rare but possible

Melissa

Melissa officinalis

Also known as: Lemon balm

Family: Labiatae

ORIGIN

Melissa is an aromatic herb native to central and southern Europe. It has been used as a medicinal herb in the treatment of melancholy and heart problems for thousands of years. Commercial production of the oil is carried out mainly in France.

THERAPEUTIC PROPERTIES

This is a sweet, calming oil. Its main action is on the nervous system and it is useful for treating many symptoms with a nervous origin. It may be used in massage blends or bath oils, and although it is expensive, just one or two drops can transform an essential oil blend. Melissa combines particularly well with citrus oils, chamomile, geranium, lavender, marjoram and rose.

Melissa's calming yet uplifting effect is very useful in the treatment of stress headaches and migraines. It is especially appropriate when the headache is associated with tension in the neck and shoulders. Melissa combines well with chamomile to treat neuralgia and any nerve pains in the body. It can be combined with rosemary or bergamot to relieve brain fatigue from over-concentration and is also good for treating depression, hysteria and anxiety.

The antispasmodic properties of melissa have a calming effect on the heart. It reduces palpitations and panic attacks and is appropriate where overwork and overstimulation have weakened the heart and caused high blood pressure. Combine it with marjoram and use in the bath and for massage. The antispasmodic properties are also helpful for painful periods.

Melissa also has an important action on the digestive system. It is a calminative to relieve flatulence, colic, dyspepsia and so on, and can also help to relieve nausea.

The cooling effect of melissa relieves fevers, especially where restlessness

METHOD OF EXTRACTION

Melissa oil is steam-distilled from the herb. Because the yield of oil is extremely small, melissa has the reputation of being one of the most frequently adulterated essential oils. True melissa oil is very expensive.

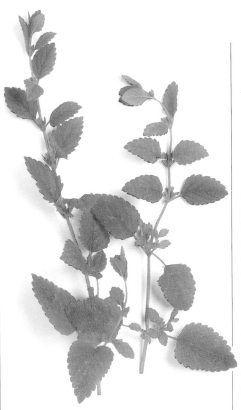

DESCRIPTION

Melissa oil is a pale yellow liquid with a pleasant lemony, fresh and sweet-herbaceous smell.

Melissa's anti-inflammatory properties are helpful for inflamed skin and allergic skin conditions. It may be used for ulceration and also for eczema, especially when stress-related. Keep it on hand as a first-aid remedy for bee or wasp stings.

PSYCHOLOGICAL PROFILE

Melissa is most appropriate if you are the type of person who appears sweet, open and extremely considerate, but do not show the darker side of your nature for fear of not being liked. You may have developed an over-concern and anxiety for the welfare of others. Although you may appear charming and cheerful, underneath there is a growing tension and frustration at not being able to express your whole self. Symptoms such as nervousness, headaches, insomnia and even heart symptoms will develop as the body suffers from these hidden tensions. Melissa will encourage you to find ways to express the whole of your personality and will enable you to relax and enjoy life to the full.

and distress are marked. Melissa can also help respiratory problems that are anxiety-related, such as asthma. To treat respiratory problems, either dilute melissa in a base oil and massage on to the chest or use in a vaporizer or essential oil burner.

MOST COMMON USES

Depression • Insomnia • Headaches
Palpitations • Colic
Inflamed skin conditions

SAFETY DATA

Non-toxic • Sensitization possible • Do not use in concentrations of more than 2%

Peppermint

Mentha piperita

Family: Labiatae

ORIGIN

Peppermint is a perennial herb that is a cultivated hybrid of other types of mint. Mint is naturalized in Europe and North America and is also cultivated throughout the world; it has been used as a medicinal herb for thousands of years, particularly as an infusion for digestive disorders. The essential oil comes primarily from the USA, although it is also produced in Europe, Russia and Morocco. The majority is used in the flavouring and toothpaste industries.

THERAPEUTIC PROPERTIES

Peppermint is cooling, refreshing, warming and stimulating. The reason for this paradox is that the body increases circulation and warms up in response to the cooling action of peppermint applied to the skin. Peppermint adds a stimulating note to many massage and bath oil blends, but use only one or two drops or the smell will overpower any other oils used. It blends particularly well with eucalyptus, lavender, lemon, pine and rosemary.

The primary action of peppermint is on the digestive system, in particular the stomach. It encourages the easy absorption of food, and can be used for any symptom of a sluggish digestion, such as indigestion and flatulence. It also helps to stop regurgitation, sour risings, belching and hiccups.

Peppermint is a digestive antiseptic and can be used to treat gastric fevers, diarrhoea and food poisoning. It is also antispasmodic, and will relieve gastric spasm and colic. It is the main oil for treating aerophagy (swallowing of air). For digestive problems, peppermint combines well with oils of fennel and orange, and may be diluted in a base oil and massaged over the abdomen.

This oil can be used to treat nausea from any cause, including morning sickness and travel sickness. Peppermint aids the digestion of fats by encouraging the flow of bile, and has a detoxifying effect on the liver.

METHOD OF EXTRACTION

The essential oil is
steam-distilled from the
flowering herb.

DESCRIPTION

Peppermint oil has a fresh, strong, minty smell with a sweet undertone. It is a pale yellow or pale green liquid.

The secondary action of peppermint is on the respiratory system. It is an expectorant and is good for treating coughs that produce yellow or green mucus. It can also be used for its antispasmodic and decongestant properties in the treatment of spasmodic coughs, asthma, bronchitis and sinusitis, and can relieve flu and head colds. Use in an essential oil burner.

Peppermint is refreshing and a general tonic of the nervous system. It will relieve nervous fatigue, and is an important oil in the treatment of migraine. It will also relieve feelings of faintness or hysteria. Its analgesic and stimulating properties make peppermint an effective treatment for neuralgia and muscular pains. Combined with lavender, it makes an excellent foot bath for tired or aching feet.

Peppermint's insect-repellent and parasiticide properties can be used to eliminate fleas, scabies and ringworm. It is a useful deodorant, and makes a good mouthwash for bad breath.

PSYCHOLOGICAL PROFILE

Peppermint is appropriate for times of transition, when one phase of life is completed and a new one about to begin, such as when changing schools or adapting to a new lifestyle. You may know that you need to leave a job or a relationship or move house, but do not yet know which direction to take. Using peppermint will help you to make a break with the past and strengthen your resolve and courage to take the next step.

OTHER VARIETIES

Spearmint oil (*Mentha spicata*) is milder and sweeter than peppermint but shares similar properties.

MOST COMMON USES

Indigestion • Nausea • Muscle pains
Coughs and colds • Deodorant

SAFETY DATA

Non-toxic externally • Do not use in cases of cardiac fibrillation
Do not use in concentrations of more than 3%

Basil

Ocimum basilicum

Family: Labiatae

ORIGIN

There are many varieties of the herb basil growing throughout the world, and all have a long tradition of use in cooking and as a herbal medicine. In Ayurvedic medicine basil is an important treatment for respiratory problems, such as coughs, asthma and bronchitis, and also as an antidote to poisonous snake bites. In Western herbal medicine it is used as a cooling herb and nerve tonic. Essential oil production mainly occurs in France, Egypt, eastern Europe and the USA.

THERAPEUTIC PROPERTIES

Basil is a very useful essential oil but there is concern about possible toxicity when using it for prolonged periods of time, so use it in moderation and only for relatively short periods, such as three weeks. It may be used in steam inhalations, and in small amounts in massage and bath oil blends. It combines particularly well with bergamot, chamomile, clary sage, geranium, lavender, lemongrass, marjoram and rose.

The main action of basil oil is on the nervous system; it is an excellent nerve tonic and has a balancing, reviving and strengthening effect. Being a balancing oil, it is both relaxing and uplifting, with an overall restorative result. It can be used to relieve brain fatigue, nervousness, anxiety, depression, tension headaches and nervous insomnia.

Where sexual problems are the result of tension, debility and overwork, the tonifying and restorative action of basil can be of help. Use in a massage, in the bath or by burning in the room. Basil can be used to treat absent or very scanty periods, especially when this is due to debility and stress. The anti-spasmodic properties of basil make it useful to treat menstrual cramp; dilute the oil and massage over the abdomen.

Basil also has a beneficial action on the digestive system, particularly the small intestine. It will relieve flatulence

METHOD OF EXTRACTION

Basil essential oil is produced by steam distillation of the flowering herb.

DESCRIPTION

The oil has a sweet, spicy, green and slightly balsamic odour and is colourless or a pale yellow colour.

and is especially good where digestive disorders are the result of nervous tension, such as nervous indigestion. The antiseptic and antispasmodic properties of basil make it useful for treating gastro-enteritis and other intestinal infections. Dilute in a base oil and massage in over the abdomen.

Basil can be used to treat spasmodic respiratory conditions such as coughs. It is also said to help restore the sense of smell – use in a steam inhalation. Basil oil is useful for debility following a prolonged fever or for lingering colds and catarrh.

Basil may be used to treat muscular weakness and muscular aches and pains. Use as a rubbing oil or compress. Basil may also be used to treat gout and rheumatism.

In first-aid treatment basil may be used to relieve wasp stings and insect bites. It also acts as a successful insect repellent.

PSYCHOLOGICAL PROFILE

Basil is appropriate if you have worn yourself out by overwork, particularly by mental effort or in a high-stress working environment. People who need basil have pushed themselves to the point where they are exhausted and their nervous system is over-wrought. Basil will help to strengthen and calm you.

OTHER VARIETIES

Of the many varieties of basil, only two chemotypes are generally used to produce essential oil – French basil and exotic basil. Of these French basil is pre-ferable for use in aromatherapy as it is less toxic and less likely to cause sensitization and irritation than the exotic type.

MOST COMMON USES

Nervous debility • Mental fatigue
Loss of sense of smell • Catarrh

SAFETY DATA

Non-irritant in dilution • Possible carcinogenic components – use in moderation
Do not use in concentrations of more than 2% • Avoid in therapeutic doses during pregnancy

Marjoram

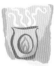

Origanum marjorana, syn. M. hortensis

Also known as: Sweet marjoram

Family: Labiatae

ORIGIN

This well-known culinary herb originated in the eastern Mediterranean and is now cultivated in central and southern Europe and North Africa. It has been used as a medicinal herb for thousands of years, and was a particular favourite of the Ancient Greeks. In herbal medicine marjoram is valued for its restorative, warming and relaxing properties.

THERAPEUTIC PROPERTIES

A warming and relaxing oil, marjoram makes an excellent addition to any massage blend or bath oil where a relaxing and calming effect is desired. It blends particularly well with bergamot, cypress, eucalyptus, geranium, lavender, orange and rosemary.

Marjoram tonifies the circulatory system, having a general vaso-dilatory effect. It can be used in the treatment of high blood pressure and narrowing of the arteries.

The sedative properties of marjoram make it good for treating anxiety, insomnia and nervous debility. It is said to be an anaphrodisiac – that is, it reduces the sexual impulse. It also has analgesic properties useful for headaches and migraines, especially those caused by stress. Its analgesic and warming properties suggest its use in the treatment of sinus pains and head colds and make it a good addition to an oil blend for the treatment of muscle pains, sprains, strains, rheumatism, arthritis, over-exertion and so on. Try combining it with eucalyptus or rosemary and use as a bath or massage oil or compress.

Marjoram is very effective at relieving painful periods, working best if massaged into the abdomen. It is also an important oil in the treatment of PMT, especially with feelings of anxiety, weariness and irritability. Sweet marjoram is safe to use externally at normal dilutions during pregnancy.

METHOD OF EXTRACTION

The essential oil is steam-distilled from the dried flowering herb.

Marjoram is an antispasmodic, alleviating colic, flatulence and dyspepsia. It also acts as a mild laxative by stimulating and strengthening intestinal peristalsis.

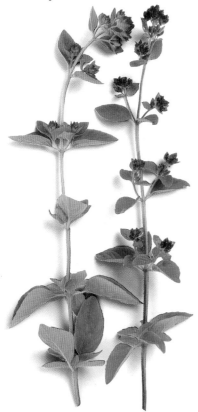

DESCRIPTION

Marjoram oil is a pale yellow or pale amber liquid with a warm and spicy, slightly camphoraceous smell.

PSYCHOLOGICAL PROFILE

Marjoram will be most appropriate if you have become exhausted and stressed as a result of overwork. You may suffer from insomnia and find it difficult to relax, and you may have thrown yourself into work as a compensation for unexpressed creative outlets or sexual activity. Eventually, enjoying life and relaxing becomes difficult. Using marjoram will allow you to relax and will open up the possibilities of a more fulfilling and enjoyable life.

OTHER VARIETIES

There are many different varieties of marjoram and oregano, and there is much confusion between them. Other varieties that are available as essential oils include oregano (*Origanum vulgare*) and Spanish oregano (*Thymus capitus*). While all varieties have therapeutic properties, both of these are skin irritants and it is advisable to use only sweet marjoram in aromatherapy.

SAFETY DATA

Non-toxic externally • Non-irritant • Non-sensitizing

Geranium

Pelargonium graveolens

Also known as: Rose geranium, geranium Bourbon, Pelargonium

Family: Geraniaceae

ORIGIN

A native of South Africa, Pelargonium graveolens *was exported to Europe in the late seventeenth century. There the pelargoniums were hybridized, later to be re-exported during the nineteenth century to the French and British colonies.*

The essential oil was first distilled in France in the early nineteenth century; today the main areas of production are Réunion, China and Egypt. Geranium is one of the most important perfumery oils.

THERAPEUTIC PROPERTIES

Geranium is a cooling and moistening oil, good where heat and dryness are present. It is calming but not necessarily sedative, as it also has an uplifting and strengthening effect. Geranium is a balancing oil, regulating in effect rather than overly sedative or stimulating. A versatile oil, it makes a fragrant addition to many blends for massage and the bath; complementary oils are bergamot, lavender, lemon, marjoram, neroli, orange, palmarosa, rose and sandalwood.

The action of geranium on the nervous system is calming and cooling, which makes it useful for treating restlessness and anxiety. It is one of the most important oils for treating menopausal symptoms including hot flushes and vaginal dryness. Add it to baths and massage oils.

Its calming effect makes geranium helpful in treating palpitations and panic attacks; it is particularly appropriate for people who wake at night feeling hot and panicky and experiencing palpitations.

The cooling properties of geranium can help to relieve symptoms arising from heat in the abdomen. These may include either constipation with dryness, or burning, yellow or offensive diarrhoea. Geranium is an effective treatment for dysentery or

METHOD OF EXTRACTION

Geranium oil is contained in glands in the leaves and green stems, from which it is steam-distilled. Harvesting occurs within a few days of the start of the flowering period, when the leaves develop a pronounced rosy scent.

gastroenteritis. In the treatment of diarrhoea it should be diluted in a base oil and massaged into the abdomen, or used as a compress over the abdomen. Its anti-inflammatory properties can help treat gastritis or peptic ulcers. It is also appropriate for cystitis with burning urination; add a few drops to the bath.

DESCRIPTION

The oil has a powerful, sweet, green, floral smell with a fruity-minty undertone. It is a pale green to olive-green liquid.

for dry or oily skin types, and is a useful antiseptic and anti-inflammatory in the treatment of acne. Its soothing properties make it appropriate for dry, inflamed skin; combine with chamomile or melissa in the treatment of dry eczema. Geranium may be applied to the skin as a lotion or compress or used in a facial steam.

The analgesic properties of geranium can help to relieve the pain of neuralgia and shingles. Use it in a massage blend or bath oil or as a compress.

Geranium has an excellent reputation in skin care and is a popular ingredient of many creams and lotions. It has a balancing effect on the sebum secretion, making it suitable

PSYCHOLOGICAL PROFILE

Geranium is appropriate if you are finding it difficult to let go of your past achievements and have become congested and 'stuck', fearful to continue to the next stage of your life. You may have lost confidence in the natural flow of life and become fearful, irritable and defensive. Geranium will help to relieve these feelings and will refresh and relax you, enabling you to move on and enjoy life again.

MOST COMMON USES

Anxiety • Hot flushes • Palpitations
Diarrhoea • Acne • Dry, inflamed skin

SAFETY DATA

Non-toxic • Non-irritant in dilution • Sensitization rare but possible

Pine

***Pinus sylvestris* (and other varieties)**

Also known as: Scots pine

Family: Pinaceae

ORIGIN

Scots pine is native to Eurasia and is also cultivated in the USA, Europe and Scandinavia. The needles have been used medicinally for hundreds of years, to relieve nervous exhaustion, for rheumatism, and by the Native Americans as an insect repellent. Pine has one of the largest productions of any essential oil. It is used extensively in disinfectants, detergents, insecticides and paint manufacture, in the paper industry and in perfumery, especially for bath crystals and soaps.

THERAPEUTIC PROPERTIES

Pine has a refreshing and 'opening' effect. Of medium temperature, it can be used for either hot or cold conditions. It may be added to massage and bath oils and also is excellent in steam inhalations. Pine combines particularly well with cedarwood, eucalyptus, juniper, lavender, lemon, marjoram and tea tree. Pine has a reviving effect on the nervous system and can be used to treat nervous exhaustion and poor concentration.

The main action of pine is on the respiratory tract – it is a powerful respiratory antiseptic and is also a decongestant. It has a strengthening effect on the lungs and can be used to treat bronchial infections, such as bronchitis, asthma, flu, coughs and colds. It will clear mucus from the chest and throat and catarrh from the sinuses. Combine with cypress to relieve the symptoms of hayfever.

The antiseptic properties of pine also have an beneficial effect on the urinary system, especially when used in the bath. It is a useful oil for treating urinary infections, such as urethritis, cystitis, pyelitis and prostatitis. Combine with eucalyptus or thyme to treat both urinary infections and venereal infections, such as non-specific urethritis (NSU).

METHOD OF EXTRACTION

Pine oil for aromatherapy use is steam-distilled from the needles. The heartwood of the pine tree is also distilled to produce turpentine. Distillation occurs mainly in the USA and Eastern Europe.

DESCRIPTION

Pine oil has a fresh, sweet, balsamic smell. It is a colourless or pale amber liquid.

This is a pleasant oil to add to the bath to ease aches and pains after a tiring day. It may also be used in compresses or massage oils to treat rheumatism, arthritis, sprains and strains.

Pine is a parasiticide against scabies and lice. It is also a good deodorant – use it as a footbath to treat smelly feet.

PSYCHOLOGICAL PROFILE

Pine is appropriate if you have a strong tendency to feel guilty. You may have been repressed as a child and punished for having a rebellious spirit or non-conformist attitudes. You may come from a strongly religious background, expecting divine retribution for your sins. This type of early experience will tend to make you fearful of enjoyment and to negate inner feelings that may cause conflict. This can produce a tendency to rigidity and self-punishment, and on the physical level induce tension and a tight chest. Using pine will help to break through all types of rigidity and will enable you to reconnect with your own sensitivity, affording you greater enjoyment and happiness in life.

OTHER VARIETIES

Other varieties of pine that are available as an essential oil include dwarf pine (*Pinus pumilio* or *P. mugo*) and also longleaf pine (*P. palustris*). Dwarf pine should not be used in aromatherapy as it is a skin irritant and common sensitizer. Longleaf pine is the most common source of turpentine and is frequently used in the USA. It shares very similar therapeutic properties with Scots pine.

MOST COMMON USES

Decongestant • Bronchitis
Hayfever • Urinary infections
Rheumatism

SAFETY DATA

Non-toxic • Do not use in dilutions of more than 3% • Sensitization possible

Black pepper

Piper nigrum

Family: Piperaceae

ORIGIN

The pepper plant is a trailing vine-like shrub native to India. Black pepper, one of the most important and oldest known spices, is the dried whole fruit. It has been used in India and China for over 4000 years as a medicine and culinary spice and became a key part of the spice trade from Asia to the West. In traditional Chinese medicine it is regarded as a treatment for malaria and a wide range of digestive disorders. The main areas of cultivation are India and Indonesia.

THERAPEUTIC PROPERTIES

Black pepper is a hot and drying oil and is suitable where there is coldness, weakness and depleted energy as it has tonifying, strengthening and stimulating properties. It may be used in massage and rubbing oils and in steam inhalations. It will irritate the skin in strong concentrations and must be very well diluted before application; do not use in concentrations of more than 0.5%. It combines particularly well with cedarwood, frankincense, juniper, lemon, marjoram, palmarosa and sandalwood.

As a stimulant to the digestive system, black pepper alleviates constipation, indigestion, flatulence, dyspepsia and a sluggish digestion. Combine with cardamom and fennel in a base oil and massage over the abdomen.

Its profoundly warming properties suggest black pepper's usefulness in treating respiratory conditions, especially if you are chilly and producing copious white mucus. It can be used in a steam inhalation to relieve head colds with these symptoms. The strongly anti-microbial properties of black pepper suggest its use in the treatment of flu and many other infections and viruses.

As a stimulant to the circulatory system, black pepper can be used in blends to treat poor circulation and cold hands and feet; combine with

METHOD OF EXTRACTION

Peppercorns are dried and crushed and then steam-distilled to produce the essential oil.

cedarwood and ginger and use as a massage oil or foot bath. It may also be used to treat chilblains.

Black pepper oil will stimulate the eliminative processes and can be used in detoxifying blends, for example, combined with juniper or rosemary. It is good in massage blends for the treatment of cellulite.

DESCRIPTION

Black pepper oil has a fresh, warm, spicy, dry-woody smell. It is a colourless or slightly green liquid.

it has a very stimulating effect on muscles it should be considered for conditions involving muscular palsy, wasting and paralysis.

PSYCHOLOGICAL PROFILE

Black pepper oil is appropriate for chilly, weak and debilitated people, who are weary and suffer from feelings of hopelessness.

The martial quality of black pepper suggests that these people may once have been fiery and energetic, but have suppressed their emotions (in particular anger) and become frustrated, introverted and weak. The use of black pepper will help to strengthen such people and develop their physical and creative energy.

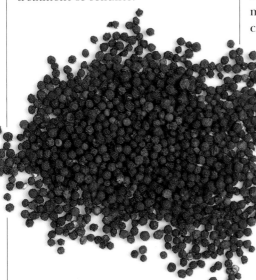

Black pepper can also be blended into an excellent rubbing oil to relieve rheumatism, sprains and aches and pains. Because

MOST COMMON USES

Sluggish digestion • Colds and flu
Cellulite • Aches and pains
Poor circulation

SAFETY DATA

Non-toxic • Non-sensitizing • Do not use in dilutions of more than 0.5%

Patchouli

Pogostemon cablin

Family: Labiatae

ORIGIN

A large-leaved herb of up to 1 m (3 ft) high, patchouli is native to tropical Asia. It has been used for centuries as an incense and also for its disinfectant and insect-repellent properties. It was traditionally incorporated into carpets and woven fabrics to give them fragrance. The distinctive and tenacious smell of patchouli has made it a popular ingredient for the perfumery industry. Distillation of the oil occurs in Asia, Europe and the USA.

THERAPEUTIC PROPERTIES

Patchouli is a stimulating and strengthening oil with astringent properties. It may be added to massage and bath oils and a little goes a long way. It may also be used to fragrance a room and is an effective deodorant. Patchouli combines well with cedarwood, geranium, neroli, orange, rose and sandalwood.

This oil has a pronounced effect on the nervous system and is an anti-depressant, but its smell is not to everyone's taste and it will only be of benefit to those who enjoy using it. It has a traditional role as an aphrodisiac and as a remedy for frigidity. It can also be used to treat nervous exhaustion, stress and anxiety.

The astringent and tonifying properties of patchouli make it a good treatment for diarrhoea – try combining it with geranium and massaging over the abdomen. Its stimulating properties can also help to relieve constipation where this is due to sluggish peristalsis and lack of muscle tone.

Patchouli shares many properties with myrrh, and can be used in steam inhalations where too much mucus is produced. It is anti-bacterial and anti-viral and may be combined with other appropriate essential oils in the treatment of many infections or viruses.

The astringent and antiseptic properties of patchouli indicate its use

METHOD OF EXTRACTION

The leaves are first lightly fermented or scalded to break the cell walls and then subjected to steam distillation to produce the essential oil.

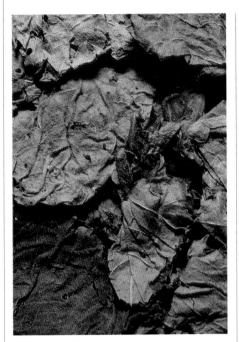

Dried patchouli leaves

DESCRIPTION

Patchouli oil has a dry, aromatic,
woody, almost musky smell. It is a thick
liquid that varies in colour from amber
to dark reddish-brown.

in the treatment of acne, oily skin, weeping sores and impetigo. It can help healthy skin tissue to regenerate and can be used to improve scars and stretch marks. Patchouli is an important oil in the treatment of ageing skin and it can help to reduce wrinkles. In skin care patchouli combines especially well with rose. It is also anti-fungal and can be used in cases of athlete's foot and other fungal infections.

PSYCHOLOGICAL PROFILE

The smell of patchouli is strongly associated with the 1960s, when it was used to evoke a mood of warmth, sexuality and a relaxed style of living. To benefit most from patchouli, you will be a person lacking in energy and drive. You may be somewhat weak, easily influenced and over-sensitive, finding it difficult to concentrate and focus on the requirements of everyday life. Using patchouli will impart a warmth and energy that will stimulate you to direct your attention, and feel more 'earthed' in your surroundings.

MOST COMMON USES

Anti-depressant • Aphrodisiac
Diarrhoea • Acne • Scars

SAFETY DATA

Non-toxic • Non-irritant • Non-sensitizing

Rose

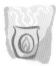

Rosa centifolia, Rosa damascena

Family: Rosaceae

ORIGIN

Roses have been used as a medicinal plant since antiquity; in the tenth century the great Persian alchemist Avicenna discovered the method for distilling rose oil. **Rosa centifolia** *(the cabbage rose) is believed to have originated in Persia and is now cultivated for extraction mainly in Morocco and France ('rose de mai' or Rose Maroc).* **Rosa damascena** *(the damask rose), probably a native of China, has been primarily cultivated in Bulgaria for the perfumery industry (otto of rose or Turkish rose). While both varieties share similar therapeutic properties,* **Rosa centifolia** *is the most commonly available for aromatherapy.*

THERAPEUTIC PROPERTIES

Rose oil is cooling, relaxing and tonifying. It is similar to bergamot, geranium and jasmine in that it decreases sympathetic nervous system activity, while at the same time strengthening the parasympathetic nervous system. This means it increases feelings of vitality and creates a sense of relaxed well-being. Rose is useful for treating a wide range of stress-related conditions in adults and hyperactivity in children. It has a low toxicity and is delightful in the bath or as a massage blend; it blends well with bergamot, chamomile, clary sage, geranium, jasmine, lavender and patchouli.

Rose oil is a great anti-depressant, helping people feel more attractive and confident. It is an excellent massage oil for scarring, and has been useful in the treatment of anorexia.

Its primary action is on reproduction and sexuality. It has a cleansing and tonifying effect on the uterus and is

METHOD OF EXTRACTION

Although the first known extract of rose was by steam distillation, the fragrance industry preferred the labour-intensive method of extraction known as enfleurage. In recent years, however, the most common form of rose extract has been the absolute made by performing solvent extraction on the rose flowers to produce a concrète. The solvent is then removed and the absolute obtained from the concrète by separation with alcohol. The essential oil is sometimes available, although it is even more costly; both are suitable for aromatherapy.

DESCRIPTION

Rose essential oil is a pale yellow liquid, while the absolute is orange-red and viscous. Both have a deep, rich and sweet rosy-floral smell.

helpful for menopausal women or those who are prone to heavy, clotted and painful periods. Its strengthening properties indicate its use for women who have a history of miscarriages. It is one of the most important oils in the treatment of PMT. As well as being a renowned treatment for infertility and frigidity in women, using rose oil increases the sperm count in men.

Rose has a tonifying effect on the vascular system and may be added to skin creams and oils to treat broken capillaries. It is particularly appropriate where symptoms of heart disease are related to stress.

On the digestive system, rose has a strengthening and detoxifying effect. Its antiseptic and anti-inflammatory properties can be used to treat gastro-enteritis and gastric ulcers. It can also relieve feelings of nausea and help to regenerate damaged intestinal walls, as

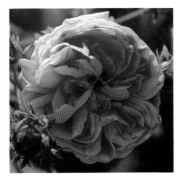

*Cabbage rose (*Rosa centifolia*)*

well as being a mild aperient useful in the treatment of chronic constipation. It has a soothing effect on the liver and gall bladder. Rose has a rejuvenating and healing effect on the skin and also has profound anti-inflammatory properties which can be used to treat dryness, inflammation, heat and itching of the skin.

PSYCHOLOGICAL PROFILE

Rose is appropriate if you have grown up with a romantic picture of love far removed from reality. You may have had the capacity for expressing yourself in a very loving way, but because reality didn't live up to your expectations you became bitter and resentful. Using rose will help to remove feelings of frustration and disappointment and will enable you to love in a way that is more understanding and tolerant of human nature.

MOST COMMON USES

Anti-depressant • Aphrodisiac • PMT
Infertility • Anti-inflammatory

SAFETY DATA

Non-toxic • Non-irritant • Non-sensitizing

Rosemary

Rosmarinus officinalis

Family: Labiatae

ORIGIN

A native of the Mediterranean countries, rosemary has been used as a medicine and a sacred herb for thousands of years. As a medicinal herb it is used primarily as a tonic for nervous debility, depression and headaches. It is also one of the classic culinary herbs.

THERAPEUTIC PROPERTIES

Rosemary is a very versatile warming and tonifying oil which has the effect of stimulating and unblocking various systems in the body. It may be used in massage blends and compresses, steam inhalations, in the bath and for room fragrancing. Rosemary combines well with many oils, especially basil, lavender, lemongrass, olibanum, orange, peppermint, petitgrain and pine.

The primary action of rosemary is on the circulatory system; it stimulates a weak heart and is useful for treating low blood pressure and cold extremities. Rosemary can also help to clear the blood vessels in cases of arteriosclerosis. Use in the bath or as a massage blend.

Rosemary increases the circulation of blood to the brain and nervous system and can help to improve memory, concentration and mental alertness, so it is a very good oil to use in a burner in any room where people are trying to concentrate. It can also be used to treat general debility, lethargy, vertigo and paralysis. It is an important remedy in the treatment of headaches and is helpful for many people who suffer with migraines.

The moving qualities of rosemary make it a good digestive tonic, promoting the flow of bile, helping to unblock an obstructed gall bladder and clearing gallstones. It is also used to treat hepatitis and jaundice.

METHOD OF EXTRACTION

Rosemary is steam-distilled from the flowers and leaves of the herb. It is produced mainly in France, Spain, Croatia, Tunisia and Morocco.

DESCRIPTION

Rosemary oil is an almost colourless or pale yellow liquid with a strong, fresh, camphoraceous and herbaceous smell.

Rosemary is an antiseptic and anti-spasmodic oil which can be employed to treat gastro-intestinal infection, painful digestion, flatulence and colic. It will alleviate diarrhoea and colitis, particularly in weak, nervous people.

Rosemary is a mild emmenagogue, and will help to relieve painful periods. Dilute in a base oil and massage over the abdomen, or add a few drops to a warm bath. It is safe to use during pregnancy at normal dilutions.

Rosemary is a beneficial oil for people prone to chronic lung conditions. It is antiseptic and tonifying and can be used to treat colds, flu and coughs. It is also one of the main detoxifying oils; combine with lavender and juniper as a massage oil to detoxify the lymphatic system.

The warming, moving qualities of rosemary make it helpful in the treatment of arthritis and rheumatism, especially when symptoms are worse in cold weather. Dilute the essential oil in a base oil to massage gently over the affected part, or apply as a compress. Rosemary will also bring relief to sprains and strains, making it a classic ingredient of sports blends. Dilute the oil and rub into painful areas. Also use before 'warming up' to help stimulate the circulation, reduce injury and improve performance.

Traditionally, rosemary has been an important treatment for problems of the hair and scalp. It stimulates the circulation to the latter and can be used to treat alopecia and dandruff. It is a parasiticide and can be used to remove lice and scabies.

PSYCHOLOGICAL PROFILE

Rosemary is an energizing oil suitable if you are cold, debilitated, weak and nervous. This may be the result of prolonged grief or of a past emotional shock that was never fully resolved, inhibiting you from freely expressing love. You may have retreated into intellectual activity as a way of avoiding emotional or physical contact and close relationships. Using rosemary will help you to regain contact with your body and unblock your emotions, enabling you to feel stronger, more 'in your body', and better able to form close emotional relationships again.

MOST COMMON USES

Poor circulation • Headaches
Aids concentration • Sprains and strains
Sports preparation • Lymphatic drainage

SAFETY DATA

Non-toxic • Non irritant in dilution • Non-sensitizing

Sage

Salvia lavandulifolia

Also known as: Spanish sage

Family: Labiatae

ORIGIN

Sage is native to the countries bordering the Mediterranean, but is now cultivated throughout the world. Like all forms of sage, Spanish sage has been used as a medicinal herb for thousands of years. It is said to promote a long life and to cure many ailments including headaches, infections, rheumatism, menstrual problems and nervous exhaustion.

THERAPEUTIC PROPERTIES

Sage is a powerful stimulant and tonifier of the nervous system, appropriate for people who are exhausted and particularly for those who have been under stress. It can help to revive people who have been studying hard for exams, and will work especially well if combined with rosemary. It can also help to build up the stamina of anaemic people, aid convalescence and relieve prolonged nervous depression. For all these conditions sage must be well diluted before use and discontinued when progress is established because of its strongly stimulating properties.

Sage oil has a tonifying effect on the circulatory system and can be used to treat low blood pressure. It can also alleviate chronic lung conditions, helping to strengthen lung tissue, and is particularly good for long-drawn-out respiratory conditions such as chronic bronchitis. It is beneficial for people who are prone to recurrent colds and flu as it will help to strengthen immunity and vitality.

In very small doses sage is anti-spasmodic and can be used to treat indigestion and dyspepsia in weak, debilitated people. It will help to improve a sluggish digestive system and stimulate the appetite. It can be used to relieve diarrhoea.

Sage has an important action on the female reproductive system and can regulate menstrual periods. Its antispasmodic properties will help to relieve painful periods if it is very well

---

METHOD OF EXTRACTION

Spanish sage oil is steam-distilled from the wild herb, which grows mainly in Spain.

DESCRIPTION

*A pale yellow liquid, Spanish sage oil
has a fresh, herbaceous and
camphoraceous smell.*

diluted. It also has a regulatory effect on hormonal problems during the menopause, and is particularly useful in relieving hot flushes and excessive perspiration; use in the bath or in a massage blend. Sage oil should never be used during pregnancy as it can stimulate uterine contractions, nor when breastfeeding as it will tend to reduce the flow of milk.

The stimulating properties of sage can be used to relieve muscular aches and pains, rheumatism and arthritis. Use in a massage blend or a compress.

Sage is an important remedy in the treatment of glandular disorders. It has a stimulating effect on the lymphatic system and can be helpful in cases of swollen glands, particularly when associated with general debility, and of benefit in cases of glandular fever and post-viral syndrome.

This oil makes an excellent mouth wash for gingivitis, receding or bleeding gums and mouth ulcers. It can also be used as a gargle for inflamed throats. Sage's astringent properties can be used to treat oily skin and hair, and it is an effective treatment for dandruff.

PSYCHOLOGICAL PROFILE

Sage is suitable if you have an undermined constitution resulting from a prolonged period of overwork or of living in an overstressed situation. In the past you may have been a high achiever and had plenty of energy, but you have become 'burnt out'. You will feel constantly tired and depressed. Using sage will help to strengthen your vitality so that you regain your energy and enjoyment in life.

OTHER VARIETIES

Common sage (*Salvia officinalis*) is also available as an essential oil, but it is high in thujone which can cause epilepsy and muscular spasm, so should be avoided.

MOST COMMON USES

Debility • Recurrent colds and flu
Hot flushes • Excessive perspiration
Gum disease • Oily skin and hair

SAFETY DATA

Non-irritant in dilution • Non-sensitizing • Do not use in pregnancy
Not to be used by people with epilepsy

Clary sage

Salvia sclarea

Family: Labiatae

ORIGIN

This distinctive variety of sage originated in the countries bordering the Mediterranean. It is an impressive plant, growing to 60–90cm/2–3ft high, with tall flower spikes rising above hairy leaves. Clary sage has been used for hundreds of years in the treatment of eye problems and digestive disorders. It is also used to flavour muscatel wine in Germany and vermouth in France. It is a classic ingredient of fine perfumes and colognes.

THERAPEUTIC PROPERTIES

Clary sage has a tonifying, warming and sedating effect; used in small amounts, it can create feelings of well-being and calmness. At the same time it will gently stimulate and strengthen the body's vitality, which makes it an excellent oil to use during convalescence and to treat depression, weakness and debility.

This oil must be well-diluted and used in moderation because it can cause drowsiness. It should be avoided when drinking alcohol as it can exaggerate the feeling of intoxication. It is excellent in massage and bath oil blends and is also pleasant to use in an essential oil burner. It combines particularly well with cardamom, coriander, geranium, jasmine, lavender, lemon, rose and sandalwood.

A renowned anti-depressant, clary sage lifts the spirits and is excellent for treating nervous tension, post-natal depression and many stress-related diseases. It can be used during the recuperative period following a breakdown and acts as an aphrodisiac where frigidity or impotence are clearly connected to stress and tension. The benefits of clary sage in treating depression and other nervous system disorders can be greatly enhanced by blending it with other appropriate oils, such as jasmine, sandalwood and geranium.

Clary sage has a tonifying effect on the female reproductive system and can strengthen a weak uterus. It will

METHOD OF EXTRACTION

The flowering tops of the herb are steam-distilled.

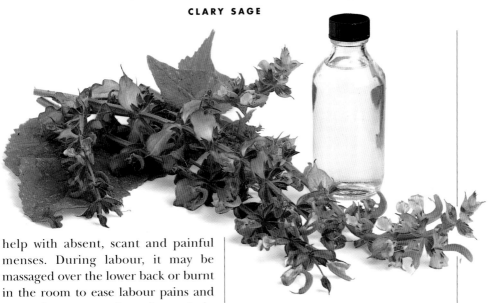

help with absent, scant and painful menses. During labour, it may be massaged over the lower back or burnt in the room to ease labour pains and strengthen contractions. It can help ease feelings of stress and nervous tension during the menopause and will also relieve excessive perspiration associated with hot flushes.

Clary sage is an effective muscle relaxant and will relieve painful muscles and muscle strain. It has hypotensive properties and can be used to treat high blood pressure, especially when this is caused by stress. It is also antispasmodic and can be used to treat asthma (especially when this is stress-related) and spasmodic coughs.

MOST COMMON USES

Anti-depressant • Convalesence
Stress and nervous tension
Painful periods

DESCRIPTION

Clary sage has a rich, bitter-sweet and herbaceous smell that is very tenacious. It is a colourless, pale yellow or pale green liquid.

PSYCHOLOGICAL PROFILE

Clary sage is appropriate if you are a nervous, fearful person who has become run down and debilitated and may lack the will to carry on. A family history of depression and hardship is likely, and as a child you may have been subjected to a lot of negativity and pessimism. Using clary sage will encourage energy and optimism for life.

SAFETY DATA

Non-toxic • Non-irritant in dilution • Non-sensitizing

Sandalwood

Santalum album

Also known as: East Indian sandalwood

Family: Santalaceae

ORIGIN

Sandalwood trees are found throughout India, though the main cultivation occurs in the southern states. The sandalwood tree is a root parasite, drawing mineral nutrients from its host. Sandalwood has been used for thousands of years to make carved sacred and decorative objects, and in powdered form as a fragrant incense. It is an important remedy in Ayurvedic and traditional Chinese medicine, and is renowned for removing the 'evil winds' that cause disease. In perfumery, it is an excellent and fixative. The essential oil is produced by the heartwood of mature trees and there used to be serious concern that more sandalwood trees were being harvested than replanted. In recent years the Indian government has intervened to ensure that there is an active programme of replanting.

THERAPEUTIC PROPERTIES

Sandalwood combines relaxing and restorative properties and is a cooling oil that has a pronounced effect on both physical and emotional problems. Because of its calming effect on the brain, it was traditionally used as an aid to meditation; it will also help to quieten a restless body and soothe the nervous system. Sandalwood combines well with rose to calm anxiety; other oils it blends well with include bergamot, cedarwood, jasmine, palmarosa, vetiver and ylang ylang. The combination of jasmine, rose and sandalwood is known as angel oil, which can be worn as a perfume and is said to help develop contact with your spirit guides.

This oil is one of the most renowned aphrodisiac oils, particularly for men. In Chinese medicine it is said to strengthen the yang. A massage with sandalwood in a base oil will enhance feelings of physical enjoyment.

METHOD OF EXTRACTION

Sandalwood oil is steam-distilled from the heartwood of the tree. There are four grades, the finest used in perfumery being Mysore sandalwood. The majority of sandalwood oil is known as Agmarked Sandalwood Oil, which is guaranteed to conform to Indian government standard.

Sandalwood is one of the main oils for treating genito-urinary tract infections, including cystitis, leucorrhoea, gonorrhoea, non-specific urethritis (NSU) and other venereal infections. It is antiseptic and encourages the body to clear out pus and infective organisms. It may be used in the bath to cure any thick, sticky discharge.

The cooling properties of sandalwood are effective for soothing inflamed mucous membranes and lung tissue, while its decongestant and antiseptic properties are beneficial in the treatment of bronchitis, laryngitis and any chronic respiratory tract infection. It may be used as a rubbing oil or as an inhalation. Sandalwood is also appropriate for any hot and painful digestive symptoms, including diarrhoea and dysentery. It will help to soothe an inflamed gall bladder.

In cosmetics and skin care, sandalwood has been in use for centuries. It

DESCRIPTION

Sandalwood oil has a long-lasting soft, deep, sweet and woody smell. It is a yellow or brownish viscous liquid.

has emollient and anti-inflammatory properties that are extremely soothing for dry, itching and inflamed skin. It is also mildly astringent and may be used on oily skin. It may be used in a cream or lotion or as a compress.

PSYCHOLOGICAL PROFILE

Sandalwood is appropriate if you feel stuck in your life, or constantly experience repeating patterns. You may approach life in a rational, intellectual way without this being balanced by the intuitive, feeling side of your nature. Your mind may go over the same episodes in your life until eventually you become confused and further from any solutions. Using sandalwood enables you to come up with fresh solutions and actions. It helps to create a wider vision of life.

MOST COMMON USES

Aphrodisiac • Meditation • Cystitis
Venereal infections • Chronic coughs
Dry skin • Weeping eczema

SAFETY DATA

Non-toxic • Non-irritant • Non-sensitizing

Clove

Syzygium aromaticum, syn. Eugenia caryophyllata

Family: Myrtaceae

ORIGIN

Clove trees originated in Asia and have been cultivated for at least 2000 years. The flower buds are dried to produce the spice we know as cloves, an important part of the spice trade since the sixteenth century. Today the main centres of cultivation are Zanzibar, Madagascar and Indonesia. Preparations of clove have been used medicinally for thousands of years to treat skin infections and infestations, digestive disorders and toothache.

THERAPEUTIC PROPERTIES

Clove is a warming and stimulating oil. It is a powerful antiseptic and highly appropriate for use in infectious diseases and the treatment of septic wounds and ulcers. It also aids the formation of scar tissue. When using clove oil on the skin it must be very well diluted or it may be an irritant; do not use in dilutions stronger than 2% and do a patch test on a small area of skin first. It is a useful addition to a room spray for fumigating a room – combine it with other strongly antiseptic oils such as bergamot, eucalyptus, lavender and thyme.

Cloves also have anti-neuralgic properties, hence the oil's well-known use for soothing the pain of toothache or an abscess. To relieve toothache, half-fill an eggcup with warm water, mix in two drops of clove oil, soak a small piece of cotton wool in the dilution and then place against the painful tooth.

Clove has anti-rheumatic and pain-relieving properties beneficial in the treatment of rheumatism, arthritis and muscular sprains and strains. Dilute well and use in a rubbing oil.

Its stimulating action makes clove an appropriate addition to oils such as rosemary for stimulating the memory and concentration. Use in an essential oil burner. Its warming and stimulating

---

METHOD OF EXTRACTION

Clove essential oil is water-distilled from the clove buds. Essential oils are also distilled from the leaves and stems but these are more toxic than clove bud oil and should not be used for aromatherapy.

---

properties also make it aphrodisiac. Clove has antispasmodic and carminative properties and can be of use in relieving flatulence, dyspepsia and diarrhoea from a chill. Dilute well in a base oil and massage over the abdomen. Its warming and antiseptic action means it is a good treatment for colds, flu and chills. It will also help to strengthen the immune system.

Clove is a useful insect repellent and parasiticide. It is of particular use against scabies; combine with cedarwood, cinnamon and lemon in a base oil and apply to the skin. To eliminate fleas and moths, combine with eucalyptus, lavender and lemon and use in a plant spray.

PSYCHOLOGICAL PROFILE

Clove is appropriate if you are generally a cheerful, outgoing and optimistic person but have been brought down by an illness, infection or trauma. You may have been suffering with a recurrent or painful condition for some time and are now becoming increasingly despondent and fed up.

DESCRIPTION

Clove oil is a pale yellow or straw-coloured liquid. The smell is strong, spicy and woody with a fruity, fresh top note.

Using clove will help to impart a sense of warmth and cheerfulness and restore your sense of optimism and enjoyment of life.

MOST COMMON USES

Infectious diseases • Toothache
Parasiticide • Insect repellent

SAFETY DATA

Non-toxic externally • Do not use in concentrations of more than 2%

Thyme

Thymus vulgaris

Also known as: Common thyme,
Red thyme (oil), White thyme (oil)

Family: Labiatae

ORIGIN

Thyme is native to Mediterranean Europe and is widely grown as a culinary herb. It has also been used as a medicinal herb for thousands of years, primarily as an antiseptic for respiratory and digestive disorders.

THERAPEUTIC PROPERTIES

Thyme oil is hot, pungent and stimulating. It is a powerful germicide, effective against many types of bacteria, viruses and fungi. It may be used in massage blends but can be an irritant, so do not use in concentrations of more than 3% and do a test on a small area of skin before use. Thyme may also be added to the bath, but it can irritate mucous membranes so should not be used in concentrations of more than 1% in bath oils. Add it to other strongly antiseptic oils such as clove, eucalyptus, lavender, lemon and pine and use in a room spray or burner to fumigate.

Thyme acts as a general nerve tonic and, in a similar way to rosemary, invigorates the brain and memory, making it a useful tonic for any exhausted or debilitated condition.

The primary action of thyme is on the genito-urinary tract. It is one of the most important oils in the treatment of venereal infections and has been used effectively in the treatment of non-specific urethritis (NSU), gonorrhoea, leucorrhoea and trichomonas. It is also effective against many types of urinary infections including cystitis and pyelitis. It has a stimulating effect on the menses and will help to bring on delayed periods.

Thyme oil is a very effective pulmonary antiseptic, so it is useful in treating respiratory infections, including colds, flu, coughs and especially bronchitis. It may be used in steam inhalations, as a chest rub or in an essential oil burner. It is particularly beneficial where there is debility associated with the respiratory infection. It is similar to eucalyptus in its expectorant properties and

METHOD OF EXTRACTION

Thyme oil is steam- or water-distilled from the flowering tops and leaves. Two types of thyme oil are produced from the plant: red thyme is the crude distillate, while white thyme is further redistilled or rectified.

DESCRIPTION

Red thyme oil is a reddish-brown liquid with a powerful, warm, spicy-herbaceous smell. White thyme oil has a fresh, herbaceous, green smell, sweeter and slightly milder than red thyme, and is colourless or pale yellow.

is also an antispasmodic, helpful for spasmodic coughs and asthma.

In a similar way to tea tree, thyme has been shown to be effective in combating infection and in strengthening the immune response by stimulating the production of white blood cells. It is one of the main essential oils to be used in the treatment of HIV-related diseases.

Thyme has a warming and tonifying effect on the digestive system. Its antiseptic properties make it useful in treating dysentery and gastro-enteritis. Combine with rosemary or geranium and massage into the abdomen.

Thyme has a stimulating and toning effect on the circulatory system. It may be used to treat low blood pressure and debility. It can be helpful for anaemia.

As a warming and stimulating oil, thyme can be used in massage blends and baths to ease muscle stiffness, aches, pains, rheumatism and arthritis.

Well diluted, thyme can be applied to the skin to heal infections, acne, boils and sores. It will also eliminate head and body lice and scabies.

PSYCHOLOGICAL PROFILE

Thyme is most appropriate if you tend to neglect or abuse your body. Over time you may have become weak, debilitated and prone to lingering infections and viruses. Using thyme will help to build up your immune system and clear out the ill effects, mentally and physically, of past habits.

OTHER VARIETIES

Wild thyme (*Thymus serpyllum*) has very similar properties to common thyme (*T. vulgaris*). Lemon thyme (*T. citriodorus*) and thyme 'linalol' are both milder and less toxic than common thyme and are therefore more suitable for children.

MOST COMMON USES

Venereal infections • Cystitis • Bronchitis
Infectious illnesses • Gastroenteritis
Rheumatism • Skin infections

SAFETY DATA

Do not use on hypersensitive or damaged skin
Do not use on infants under 2 years of age • Dilute well before use

Vetiver

***Vetiveria zizanoides,
syn. Andropogon muricatus***

Family: Gramineae

ORIGIN

Vetiver is a tall perennial grass related botanically to citronella, lemongrass and palmarosa. A native of India, it is cultivated for essential oil production in southern India, Indonesia, the Caribbean and South America. The grass has a practical agricultural use as the dense lacework of rootlets helps to prevent soil erosion on steep slopes during torrential tropical rains. The roots have been used in Asia for centuries for their fragrance, and are woven into aromatic matting and screens. Vetiver oil has always been in great demand by perfumers as a base note in many oriental, woody and chypre fragrances. Distillation occurs either near the area of cultivation, or the grass is exported for distillation in the USA and Europe.

THERAPEUTIC PROPERTIES

The main action of vetiver is on the nervous system and it is both sedating and strengthening in effect. It is excellent in the treatment of depression, nervous tension, debility, insomnia and many stress-related diseases, and acts as an aphrodisiac where there is a clear connection between impotence or frigidity and stress. Vetiver may be used in massage blends and the bath; it has a rather powerful smell but is very pleasant when diluted. It blends well with other anti-depressant oils, such as clary sage, jasmine, lavender, patchouli, rose, sandalwood and ylang ylang.

Vetiver stimulates the circulatory system and makes a useful massage oil for elderly or debilitated people with poor circulation. It also helps to stimulate the production of red blood cells and is thus beneficial for anaemia.

Vetiver makes a useful warming and pain-relieving rubbing oil, suitable for deep massage of muscular aches and pains, sprains, stiffness, rheumatism

METHOD OF EXTRACTION

The oil is steam-distilled from the rootlets, which are washed, dried, cut and chopped, then usually soaked again in water prior to distillation.

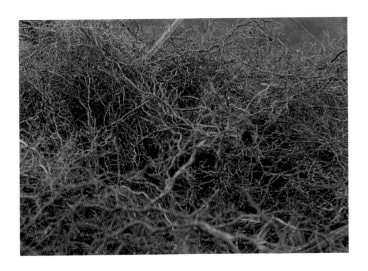

DESCRIPTION

Vetiver oil is an amber, olive or dark brown viscous liquid which has a sweet, heavy smell with a woody, earthy undertone and a lemony top note.

and arthritis. It may be added to sports oil blends and massaged into muscles before and after sports.

In skin care, vetiver helps to balance the secretion of sebum. It is also a useful antiseptic and is slightly astringent. Use it in lotions, compresses and baths for the treatment of oily skin, acne and weeping sores.

PSYCHOLOGICAL PROFILE

Vetiver is most appropriate when you are feeling emotionally overwhelmed. You may be weepy, feeling under pressure and uncertain which direction to take. It may be that you have been dominated by a particular situation or person and need to learn to make decisions for yourself. You may be leaving an institution, or relationship, or entering a different phase of your life. Using vetiver will enable you to keep calm and deal with the stress of change so that you can begin to see new opportunities and directions.

MOST COMMON USES

Anti-depressant • Aphrodisiac
Muscular aches and pains • Oily skin

SAFETY DATA

Non-toxic • Non-irritant • Non-sensitizing

Ginger

Zingiber officinale

Family: Zingiberaceae

ORIGIN

The ginger plant is native to coastal regions of India. It is a perennial herb with a tuberous rhizome root that has been used as a culinary and medicinal spice for several thousand years. It has been grown in the Caribbean since the early sixteenth century and formed an early part of the spice trade to Europe. In recent years ginger has been grown commercially in West Africa, the Far East and the Caribbean. The essential oil is used to add warmth and depth to oriental and masculine fragrances. It is also widely used as a flavouring for food and drinks.

THERAPEUTIC PROPERTIES

Ginger is a hot, moving and tonifying oil for use in cold, weak and stuck conditions. It makes an excellent warming massage or rubbing oil. It may also be used in footbaths, but as it may irritate sensitive mucous membranes it is best avoided in general bath oils. Ginger blends particularly well with cedarwood, coriander, frankincense, juniper, palmarosa, sandalwood, vetiver and all citrus oils.

One of the main areas ginger acts on is the lungs. Its tonifying qualities help chronic cold conditions in people who have a tendency to keep catching colds and flu. Ginger encourages the body to produce heat and sweat and throw off fevers, and acts as an expectorant where the mucus is white, indicating a cold condition. The moving effects of ginger help to relieve headaches caused by congestion and blocked sinuses.

The stimulating properties of ginger make it one of the most important oils for strengthening the immune system – use it in foot baths or inhalations at the beginning of winter to encourage immunity against colds and flu. It stimulates and strengthens the adrenal cortex and may be blended into a massage oil and massaged over the kidney area to improve vitality if you are cold and weak.

METHOD OF EXTRACTION

Ginger essential oil is steam-distilled from the dried rhizomes.

DESCRIPTION

The essential oil has a familiar hot, sweet, pungent and spicy odour. It is pale yellow or light amber in colour.

Ginger is an excellent oil for treating circulatory problems. It will combine well with cypress to treat chilblains, or can be used alone in a footbath to improve chronically cold feet.

One of ginger's most important uses is in treating ailments of the digestive system. It is most beneficial if you have a slow and weak digestion; it will relieve flatulence and help to improve assimilation and tone the digestive process. It will also bring relief to diarrhoea brought on by a chill.

Ginger can be used to treat arthritis and rheumatism where the symptoms are worse in cold and damp weather. It will work well if combined with peppermint and juniper in a base oil and massaged into the joints. Ginger may also be used to relieve muscle fatigue or aches and pains after over-exertion, as well as help with sprains and strains.

The strengthening and tonifying properties of ginger indicate its use as an aphrodisiac. It will work best if added to a base oil and massaged in over the kidney area.

As a first-aid remedy, ginger can help to relieve travel sickness, morning sickness and nausea. Place a couple of drops on a tissue and inhale the vapours at frequent intervals.

PSYCHOLOGICAL PROFILE

Ginger is useful if you are the type of person who is easily swayed by circumstances and frequently side-tracked. Everything has become an effort and all courses of action seem to have too many difficulties to work out well. You may feel flat, apathetic and indecisive. Using ginger oil will create a sense of determination and confidence, so that you can work through difficulties with a greater sense of your own inner power.

MOST COMMON USES

Colds and flu • General debility
Poor circulation • Weak digestion
Rheumatism • Nausea

SAFETY DATA

Non-toxic • Non-sensitizing • Non-irritant in dilution

125

Blending
Essential Oils

All essential oils can be blended to create
new combinations. Some recommendations
of oils that combine well have been given on
the previous pages, and recipes of favourite
blends are contained in this section – use the
ideas as a starting point, and experiment to
create your own blends. Most essential oils
need to be diluted in a base oil before being
applied to the skin; the following pages
give details of the best base oils to use.
Remember, blending is an art, requiring a
combination of technique and creative flair.

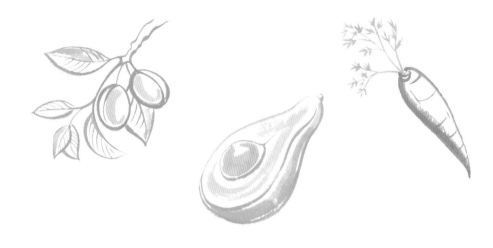

Base Oils

Base oils, or carrier oils, are used as a medium in which to dilute the essential oils before applying to the skin. There are a number of base oils that are suitable, all with slightly different properties. Use only vegetable, nut or seed oils as mineral oil tends to block the pores and is not as readily absorbed, and wherever possible buy machine-expressed or cold-pressed oils in preference to heat- or solvent-extracted oils as the former will retain more of the plant nutrients. Some organically produced oils are also available, and these are free of biocide and synthetic fertilizer residues.

Macerated oils can also make an excellent base for the addition of essential oils. These are plant oils, such as sunflower or olive, that have had a herb steeped in them so that the properties of the herb are infused into the oil.

All base oils should be as fresh as possible. Any oil that smells rancid or is more than two years old should not be used.

ALMOND OIL (SWEET)

One of the most popular of all the base oils, almond is a nearly odourless, fairly light oil that is readily absorbed by the skin. It has a soothing effect and is well tolerated by most skin types, although sensitization is possible. It makes a good general-purpose massage base. Almond oil is usually available cold-pressed, when it contains vitamins A, B1, B2, B6 and a small amount of vitamin E.

APRICOT KERNEL OIL

Apricot kernel oil is a light and odourless oil similar in properties to almond. Being light, it is suitable for applying to the face and other areas of delicate skin. It contains vitamin A and some B group vitamins.

ARNICA OIL

This is a macerated oil made with the herb *Arnica montana*, which is renowned for its therapeutic properties. It is excellent for treating bruises, bumps, contusions, aches and pains, over-exertion, backache, injuries, strains and sprains. Do not use arnica oil on broken skin.

AVOCADO OIL

Avocado is a thick green oil when cold-pressed, more viscous and pale yellow when heat-extracted. Cold-pressed avocado oil is rich in nutrients (vitamins A, B and D and lecithin) and keeps fairly well. It is excellent for dry and ageing skin. Because of its viscosity it should be used as part of a massage base blend, for example 10–25% in a lighter base oil such as almond.

CALENDULA OIL

This is a macerated oil containing the herb marigold (*Calendula officinalis*), which has excellent healing and anti-inflammatory properties. Calendula oil is suitable for any damaged skin, and especially for wounds, ulcers, bed sores, eczema, scars, and chapped and cracked skin. It will also help to prevent stretch marks during pregnancy and may be massaged on to sore nipples. It may be used on its own or blended with other base oils.

CARROT OIL

Carrot oil is a nourishing orange-coloured oil made by blending carrot extract with a vegetable oil. It is rich in beta-carotene and vitamins B, C, D and E. This oil is excellent for prematurely ageing, inflamed, damaged or scarred skin. When buying it, check that it is in fact made from carrots as commercial carrot oil is often produced from *Tagete* flowers instead. The orange colour of carrot oil can stain the skin and clothing, so allow plenty of time for the oil to be absorbed before getting dressed, or use in a partial dilution with other base oils.

COCONUT OIL

Coconut oil is solid at room temperature but liquefies at body heat, so before use melt it by warming it in your hand or on a radiator. It is traditionally used for dry skin and especially for hair and scalp treatments. You can melt the coconut oil, add the essential oils and stir before allowing the oil to set again so that you can use a little of the prepared oil as required.

COMFREY OIL

This is a macerated oil using the herb comfrey (*Symphytum officinalis*), renowned for its healing properties. Comfrey oil is excellent for treating scars, rheumatism and arthritis, aches and pains, broken bones, bruises, wounds and burns.

EVENING PRIMROSE OIL

Evening primrose oil is rich in linoleic acid and also contains gamma linoleic acid (GLA) and other vitamins and minerals. It is excellent in the treatment of eczema, psoriasis and dry and ageing skin but is rather expensive. Use as 10% or more of a base oil blend.

GRAPESEED OIL

Grapeseed is a light and odourless oil that is particularly suitable for the massage of oily skin. It contains linoleic acid and a small

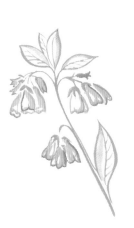
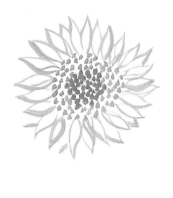
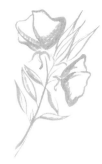

amount of vitamin E. It can be blended or used as a 100% base oil.

HAZELNUT OIL

A rich and nourishing oil that has a pleasant nutty smell. It contains oleic acid, linoleic acid, vitamins and minerals. Hazelnut oil is particularly useful for treating acne and scarred or ageing skin. It may be used as part of a blend or as a 100% base oil.

JOJOBA OIL

This is not actually an oil but a liquid wax. It is stable and keeps well, but is rather expensive. Jojoba oil combines readily with sebum and is highly penetrative. It is a balancing oil, good for treating acne and oily skin as well as dry and dehydrated skin. It is also anti-inflammatory and may be used for the treatment of eczema and psoriasis.

OLIVE OIL

As well as being a culinary oil, olive oil has been used for centuries for cosmetic and therapeutic purposes. It is particularly beneficial for treating rheumatism, aches and pains and dry or inflamed skin. Cold-pressed olive oil is rich in a number of vitamins and minerals. Because it is rather thick and green, it is more pleasant to use if diluted 10–50% with other base oils.

ST JOHN'S WORT OIL

A macerated oil made with St John's wort herb (*Hypericum perforatum*), which has antiseptic, healing and pain-relieving properties. It has the ability to soothe nerve pain and is excellent for treating sciatica, backache, neuralgia, lumbago and shingles; it may also be used for damaged skin, burns, wounds and ulcers. Good-quality St John's wort oil is traditionally made using olive oil and should be a beautiful deep red colour.

SUNFLOWER OIL

This is a pleasant, light oil that is available organically produced and cold-pressed. It is often used as the base for good-quality macerated oils. Cold-pressed sunflower oil contains vitamins A, B, D and E. It makes an excellent massage oil base.

WHEATGERM OIL

Wheatgerm is a thick, amber-coloured oil that if unrefined is naturally rich in vitamin E. It is suitable for dry, damaged, ageing or scarred skin and will help to prevent stretch marks during pregnancy. Wheatgerm oil is rather viscous so should be blended with other lighter base oils at a dilution of 10–20%. Despite the anti-oxidant properties of vitamin E, wheatgerm oil tends to deteriorate quickly so should be used within 12 months of purchase.

Essential Oil Blends

Some favourite recipes are given here for you to follow, but once you are a little more confident you should begin to experiment – it will help you to learn about the oils as well as giving you the opportunity to make a unique oil combination of your own.

BLENDING

When blending oils yourself, bear in mind the following guidelines:

- Blending is an art, and like all arts it is a combination of technique and creative flair.
- The most pleasing blend is likely to have a balance of what perfumers call 'base', 'middle' and 'top' notes. Base notes have a deep, rich smell, for example sandalwood, vetiver and ylang ylang. Middle notes include most of the floral smells such as geranium and lavender. Top notes have a light, refreshing smell such as is found in the citrus oils.
- Do not use too many essential oils in any one blend – between four and seven is usually about right.
- If you spoil a blend by a poor combination it is unlikely that you will be able to correct your mistake; it is better to start again.

- Make a record of your blends as you go along; smell, evaluate and write a comment after each addition of an oil.
- Less is more; just two drops of an essential oil can transform a blend.
- If you like a blend you are more likely to use it; be good to yourself.
- Most people find blending easier if it is done into an odourless base oil such as almond. Try using 30 ml/1 fl oz/2 tbsp of base oil. Assuming that 20 drops of essential oil is 1 ml, making a 2% massage blend will require 12 drops of combined essential oil (blends should be 1–3%).
- Make your blend in a small beaker, a tea cup or a wide-necked bottle.
- Once complete, store your blend in a glass bottle and label with the details of the mixture (or a name) and the date that you made it.

All recipes for massage blends are for 30 ml/2 tbsp. If you find you use a lot of a particular blend, just multiply the amounts accordingly.

Recipes

STIMULATING SPORTS OIL

An excellent rubbing oil to help with the warm-up process or to relieve any over-exertion after sports. Rub into areas of muscle, paying particular attention to any painful areas, before and after activity.

GINGER	**1 drop**
LAVENDER	**4 drops**
LEMONGRASS	**3 drops**
ROSEMARY	**4 drops**
VETIVER	**3 drops**

Add to a base of 10 ml/2 tsp arnica oil and 25 ml/5 tsp almond oil.

SENSUAL MASSAGE OIL – FEMININE

A delicious-smelling combination of sensual and aphrodisiac essential oils.

BERGAMOT	**2 drops**
CORIANDER	**2 drops**
JASMINE	**6 drops**
ROSE	**4 drops**
SANDALWOOD	**2 drops**

For a massage oil, add to a base of 30 ml/2 tbsp almond or sunflower oil. For a bath oil, double the amounts of the essential oils and mix with 30 ml/2 tbsp almond oil; add 10 ml/2 tsp to each bath.

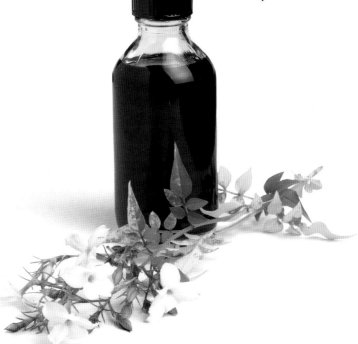

SENSUAL MASSAGE OIL – MASCULINE

A fragrant and aphrodisiac blend of essential oils excellent for a sensual massage.

CEDARWOOD	**4 drops**
FRANKINCENSE	**2 drops**
ORANGE	**2 drops**
SANDALWOOD	**8 drops**
VETIVER	**2 drops**
YLANG YLANG	**2 drops**

Add to a base of 30 ml/2 tbsp almond or grapeseed oil.

FOCUS THE MIND

An excellent aid to concentration and memory. Use when studying for exams, for example, or during meditation.

CEDARWOOD	**4 drops**
CLOVE	**1 drop**
FRANKINCENSE	**6 drops**
LEMON	**2 drops**
ORANGE	**2 drops**
ROSEMARY	**2 drops**

Add to 30 ml/2 tbsp almond oil and use as a massage oil. Alternatively, mix the essential oils into an empty 10 ml/2 tsp bottle and add a few drops at a time to an essential oil burner.

RELAXING MASSAGE/BATH OIL

A relaxing and fragrant blend of oils, this is ideal to use for general massage.

BERGAMOT	**2 drops**
GERANIUM	**4 drops**
LAVENDER	**6 drops**
MARJORAM	**4 drops**

Add these oils to 30 ml/2 tbsp almond oil for an excellent general massage oil. For a bath oil, double the amounts of the essential oils and mix with 30 ml/2 tbsp almond oil; add 10 ml/2 tsp to each bath. Mix the essential oils into an empty 10 ml/2 tsp bottle and add a few drops at a time to an essential oil burner to fragrance the room.

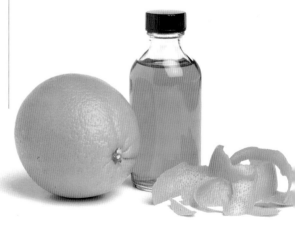

SENSITIVE SKIN OIL

A very mild and soothing, anti-inflammatory blend, useful for healing damaged or very dry or sensitive skin and eczema. This blend also makes a delightful massage oil for babies of 6 weeks old and over.

LAVENDER	**6 drops**
ROSE	**2 drops**
ROMAN CHAMOMILE	**4 drops**

Add to a mixture of 10 ml/2 tsp calendula oil and 25 ml/5 tsp almond or sunflower oil. The essential oil blend may be used in warm water as a soothing compress (half the amounts of essential oils to a bowl of warm water).

INSECT REPELLENT

Excellent for repelling mosquitoes and many other insects.

CEDARWOOD	**4 drops**
EUCALYPTUS	**2 drops**
CITRONELLA	**8 drops**
LAVENDER	**4 drops**

Add to 30 ml/2 tbsp lavender water and apply to exposed areas of skin with an atomizer. The oils may also be added to 30 ml/2 tbsp almond oil and applied to the skin, or added to an essential oil burner.

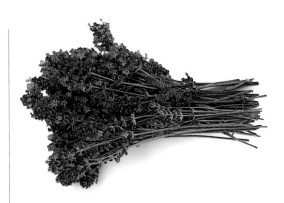

RHEUMATISM OIL

A warming blend of oils that will relieve stiffness and pain in inflamed muscles and joints. It may also be used for sprains, strains and backache.

CYPRESS	**2 drops**
GINGER	**3 drops**
JUNIPER	**4 drops**
LAVENDER	**4 drops**
PINE	**2 drops**

Add to a mixture of 10 ml/2 tsp comfrey oil and 25 ml/5 tsp almond oil and massage into painful areas. To make a bath oil, double the quantity of essential oils and add to the same mixture of base oils; add 10 ml/2 tsp to each bath. The essential oils may also be mixed in an empty bottle and 4–6 drops of the mixture added to a bowl of warm water for a compress.

STRESS-RELIEVER

A soothing and uplifting blend of essential oils guaranteed to relieve feelings of stress.

BASIL	2 drops
CLARY SAGE	4 drops
LAVENDER	4 drops
NEROLI	4 drops
PALMAROSA	2 drops

Add to 30 ml/2 tbsp almond oil as a massage oil. For a bath oil, double the quantities of essential oils and add to 30 ml/2 tbsp almond oil; add 10 ml/2 tsp to each bath. Mix the essential oils into an empty 10 ml/2 tsp bottle and add a few drops at a time to an essential oil burner to fragrance the room.

CELLULITE OIL

A detoxifying oil blend that will help stimulate the lymphatic system and break down cellulite.

BLACK PEPPER	3 drops
CYPRESS	2 drops
FRANKINCENSE	2 drops
GERANIUM	6 drops
GRAPEFRUIT	2 drops
JUNIPER	4 drops
SANDALWOOD	2 drops

Add to 30 ml/2 tbsp almond oil and massage into areas of cellulite on a daily basis.

IMMUNO-STIMULANT BLEND

A blend to stimulant the immune system and help fight off any infection, especially colds, flu or coughs.

LAVENDER	4 drops
LEMON	2 drops
PINE	4 drops
TEA TREE	6 drops
THYME	1 drop

Add to 30 ml/2 tbsp almond oil and use as a massage oil for over the kidney area or as a chest rub. Alternatively, put the blend in a 10 ml/2 tsp bottle and add 4–6 drops to a footbath or use as a steam inhalation.

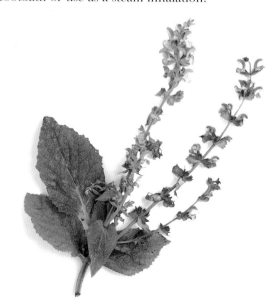

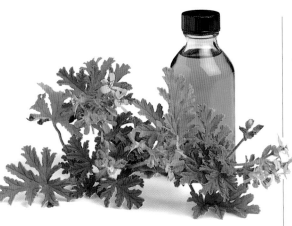

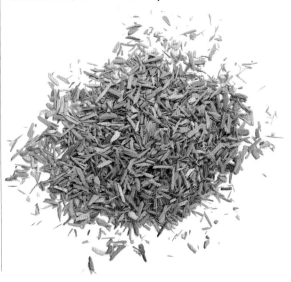

REGENERATIVE BLEND

A luxurious and rejuvenating oil suitable for prematurely ageing, tired or wrinkled skin. It will also have a tonifying effect on the whole system when you are feeling exhausted.

CEDARWOOD	**2 drops**
FRANKINCENSE	**4 drops**
JASMINE	**4 drops**
PALMAROSA	**2 drops**
SANDALWOOD	**4 drops**

Add to a mixture of 5 ml/1 tsp avocado oil and 30 ml/2 tbsp almond oil and massage into the skin. For a bath oil, the quantities of essential oil can be doubled and added to 30 ml/2 tbsp almond oil; use 10 ml/2 tsp for each bath.

FACIAL STEAM BLEND

Excellent for treating blackheads, acne and problem skin. Use as a facial steam twice a week for six weeks for best results. It also makes an excellent deep-cleansing facial steam for any skin type on an occasional basis.

BERGAMOT	**4 drops**
CHAMOMILE	**2 drops**
GERANIUM	**4 drops**
GRAPEFRUIT	**4 drops**
JUNIPER	**2 drops**
PATCHOULI	**2 drops**

Combine in a 10 ml/2 tsp dropper bottle and add 3–4 drops to a bowl of hot water for a facial steam. You can also add the essential oils to 30 ml/2 tbsp grapeseed oil and apply to the skin as a facial tonic oil.

Essential Oils and their Properties

	Acne	Allergies	Anxiety	Apathy	Blisters	Bronchitis	Bruises	Burns	Candida	Colds	Concentration	Confusion	Coughs	Cramp	Cuts	Depression	Eczema	Exhaustion	Fear	Flu	Headache
Basil			✔			✔					✔					✔		✔			
Bergamot			✔	✔							✔			✔		✔					✔
Cardamom													✔								✔
Cedarwood	✔					✔				✔			✔								
Chamomile	✔	✔	✔		✔		✔										✔		✔		✔
Cinnamon				✔					✔									✔		✔	
Clary sage			✔										✔			✔		✔			
Clove																					
Coriander				✔					✔	✔			✔					✔		✔	✔
Cypress							✔					✔	✔								
Eucalyptus						✔			✔	✔			✔							✔	✔
Fennel						✔	✔						✔	✔							
Frankincense				✔		✔					✔					✔		✔			
Geranium	✔		✔								✔					✔					
Ginger				✔		✔				✔			✔					✔		✔	
Grapefruit	✔			✔		✔				✔		✔	✔							✔	✔
Jasmine			✔										✔						✔		
Juniper	✔												✔								
Lavender	✔	✔	✔		✔		✔	✔	✔	✔					✔	✔	✔	✔	✔		✔
Lemon	✔		✔									✔	✔								
Lemongrass	✔																				
Mandarin			✔			✔										✔					
Marjoram			✔							✔				✔	✔		✔		✔		✔
Melissa		✔	✔										✔			✔	✔				✔
Myrrh	✔					✔		✔		✔			✔					✔	✔		
Neroli											✔										✔
Orange				✔														✔			
Palmarosa	✔			✔														✔			
Patchouli	✔											✔									
Pepper				✔		✔			✔						✔			✔	✔		
Peppermint				✔					✔											✔	✔
Pine						✔			✔	✔	✔	✔							✔	✔	✔
Rose			✔										✔			✔			✔		
Rosemary				✔					✔	✔			✔					✔		✔	✔
Rosewood	✔		✔							✔		✔						✔	✔		
Sage						✔							✔					✔		✔	✔
Sandalwood			✔			✔							✔				✔				
Star anise						✔				✔			✔	✔							
Tea tree	✔				✔	✔	✔	✔	✔	✔					✔				✔		
Thyme	✔	✔				✔		✔	✔	✔			✔	✔				✔	✔	✔	
Vetiver	✔													✔	✔				✔		
Ylang ylang																✔					

	Hyperactivity	Insect bites	Insect repellent	Insomnia	Irritability	Jet lag	Laryngitis	Mood swings	Muscle aches	Panic attacks	Period pains	PMT	Rheumatism	Shock	Sprains	Stress	Sunburn	Toothache	Upset stomach	Warts	Worry
Basil		✔	✔	✔				✔		✔			✔			✔					
Bergamot					✔	✔										✔					
Cardamom																			✔		
Cedarwood																					
Chamomile	✔	✔		✔						✔	✔		✔				✔	✔	✔		
Cinnamon			✔										✔								
Clary sage	✔			✔					✔			✔				✔					✔
Clove			✔															✔			
Coriander					✔			✔		✔			✔		✔						
Cypress				✔			✔	✔					✔								
Eucalyptus			✔					✔													
Fennel													✔								
Frankincense										✔											✔
Geranium				✔			✔					✔				✔					
Ginger								✔					✔		✔	✔			✔		
Grapefruit								✔													
Jasmine										✔						✔					
Juniper								✔					✔								
Lavender	✔	✔	✔	✔	✔	✔	✔	✔	✔	✔			✔	✔	✔	✔	✔		✔		✔
Lemon			✔				✔						✔							✔	
Lemongrass			✔																		
Mandarin	✔			✔												✔					✔
Marjoram			✔	✔				✔	✔	✔	✔		✔		✔	✔					
Melissa	✔	✔	✔	✔	✔					✔	✔	✔		✔		✔			✔		✔
Myrrh			✔				✔														
Neroli			✔											✔		✔					
Orange																✔					
Palmarosa																✔					
Patchouli																					
Pepper								✔					✔			✔					
Peppermint			✔			✔												✔	✔		
Pine								✔					✔			✔					
Rose							✔				✔	✔					✔	✔			
Rosemary					✔			✔					✔			✔					
Rosewood	✔			✔			✔			✔		✔		✔		✔					✔
Sage							✔	✔		✔			✔			✔					
Sandalwood				✔			✔														✔
Star anise				✔				✔		✔			✔						✔		
Tea tree		✔												✔	✔					✔	
Thyme			✔										✔			✔	✔				
Vetiver							✔	✔						✔		✔					
Ylang ylang			✔	✔						✔						✔					

Further Reading

Arctander, S., *Perfume and Flavour Materials of Natural Origin.* Elizabeth, New Jersey, USA, 1960.

Bach, E., *Heal Thyself.* C W Daniel, Saffron Walden, UK, 1931.

Barnard, J., *A Guide to the Bach Flower Remedies.* C W Daniel, Saffrol Walden, UK, 1979.

Curtis, S., Fraser, R. and Kohler, I., *Neal's Yard Natural Remedies.* Arkana, London, 1988.

Curtis S. and Fraser, R., *Natural Healing For Women.* HarperCollins, London, 1991.

Davis, P., *Aromatherapy: An A–Z.* C W Daniel, Saffron Walden, UK, 1988.

Davis, P., *Subtle Aromatherapy.* C W Daniel, Saffron Walden, UK, 1991.

Gawain, S., *Living in the Light.* Whatever Publishing, Mill Valley, California, USA.

Grieve, Mrs M., *A Modern Herbal.* Penguin, London, 1931.

Heindel, M., *The Vital Body.* Fowler, London, 1950.

Hoffman, D., *The Holistic Herbal.* Findhorn Press, Scotland, 1983.

Lawless, J., *The Illustrated Encyclopedia of Essential Oils.* Element, Shaftesbury, 1995.

Maury, M., *Marguerite Maury's Guide to Aromatherapy.* C W Daniel, Saffron Walden, 1961.

Phillips, A. and Rakusen, J., *The New Our Bodies Ourselves.* Penguin, London, 1989.

Ryman, D., *The Aromatherapy Handbook.* C W Daniel, Saffron Walden, UK, 1984.

Stein, D., *The Women's Spirituality Book.* Llewellyn Publications, St Paul, Minnesota, USA, 1987.

Tisserand, M., *Aromatherapy for Women.* Thorsons, London, 1985.

Tisserand, R., *The Art of Aromatherapy.* C W Daniel, Saffron Walden, UK, 1977.

Tisserand, R. and Balacs, T., *Essential Oil Safety.* Churchill Livingstone, Edinburgh, 1975.

Worwood, V., *The Fragrant Pharmacy.* Bantam, London, 1990.

Valnet, J., *The Practice of Aromatherapy.* C W Daniel, Saffron Walden, UK, 1980.

Useful Addresses

The Neal's Yard Remedies range of essential oils can be obtained in many parts of the world. If you have any difficulty in locating the oils, contact the UK head office for details of your nearest outlet:

Head office: 26–34 Ingate Place
                London SW8 3NS
                Tel: 0171 498 1686
                Fax: 0171 498 2505

Mail order: 5 Golden Cross
                Cornmarket Street
                Oxford OX1 3EU
                Tel/fax: 0186 524 5436

Neal's Yard Remedies shops and franchises:
15 Neal's Yard, Covent Garden, London
    WC2H 9DP (Tel: 0171 379 7222)

Chelsea Farmers Market, Sydney Street,
    London SW3 6NR (Tel: 0171 351 6380)
9 Elgin Crescent, London W11 2JA
    (Tel: 0171 727 3998)
5 Golden Cross, Cornmarket Street, Oxford
    OX1 3EU (Tel: 0186 524 5436)
126 Whiteladies Road, Clifton, Bristol
    BS8 2RP (Tel: 0117 946 6034)
68 Chalk Farm Road, Camden, London
    NW1 8AN (Tel: 0171 284 2039)
The Glades Shopping Centre, Bromley, Kent
    BR1 1DD (0181 313 9898)
2A Kensington Gardens, Brighton BN1 4AL
    (Tel: 0127 360 1464)
31 King Street, Manchester M2 6AA
    (Tel: 0161 831 7875)
26 Lower Goat Lane, Norwich, NR2 1EL
    (Tel: 0160 376 6681)

Aromatherapy organizations around the world:

UK: Aromatherapy Organizations Council, 3 Latymer Close, Braybrooke,
            Market Harborough, Leicester LE16 8LN (Tel: 0185 843 4242)
            An umbrella organization with a large list of practitioners.
            (Send an A5 s.a.e. for information.)

USA: NAHA (National Association of Holistic Aromatherapists), 219 Carl Street,
            San Francisco, California CA 94117 (Tel: 415 564 6785)
            An umbrella organization with a large list of practitioners.

Australia: Association of Massage Therapists, 18a Spit Road, Mosman, NSW 2088
            (Tel: 969 8445)

            Australasian College of Natural Therapies, 620 Harris Street, Ultimo, NSW 2007
            (Tel: 02 212 6699)

Index